The Magic Pill For The Perfect Body

By

Gatis Jerins

Copyright © 2025 Gatis Jerins

ISBN: tbc

All rights reserved, including the right to reproduce this book, or portions thereof in any form. No part of this text may be reproduced, transmitted, downloaded, decompiled, reverse engineered, or stored, in any form or introduced into any information storage and retrieval system, in any form or by any means, whether electronic or mechanical without the express written permission of the author.

Chapters

1.	It sucks! But wait?	1
2.	Are you the right person for Magic Pill?	9
3.	Be aware!	13
4.	Me and pill	33
5.	The Magic Pill	38
6.	Magic Pill double-strength supplement	59
7.	How you look and feel being addicted	78
8.	Have you been diagnosed correctly?	84
9.	How to swallow a pill	88
10.	Magic Pill side-effects	102
11.	The pill did magic! What next?	117
12.	Summary	124

It sucks! But wait?

It sucks to be fat! I'm sick of being out of shape! I'm unhappy and confused to be at that point where I'm unable to tie up my own shoelaces! I'm so, so tired of working on my dream body, but all I get is failure after failure! You have done that a hundred times and always had the same unsuccessful result. Sound familiar?

Congratulations, you have found the right reading material. What would you say if I told you I know a secret magic pill for you to get your perfect body? Everyone wants that simple, effortless way to get that dream physique. So, here I am with a solution to your problem. I promise, magic pills exist, and they work miracles. But keep an open mind because it's a different-looking pill than you might think. In this book, I'll give you all the information you need through guided chapters. Now it's time for you to promise me that you will follow my directions for that magical pill, and with it, you will obtain your perfect dream body. It's going to be a team effort, with me directing and you acting, but first, sit tight for an eye-opening read.

This self-help book was exactly what I needed when I was starting my perfect body journey. Knowing little about how to get to my dream body, I desperately wanted this pill. I had no idea something like that existed. After discovering this magical pill, I felt like I saw the light at the end of the tunnel.

You will have exclusive directions like what the magical pill looks like, how to choose the strength of the pill, what supplements you will need for double strength, how to swallow that pill, what side-effects you will face, and what to do next after the pill does its magic. Unfortunately for me, I didn't have all this information in one place. This book will save you a lot of time and solve one or more of your problems. Remember all those wasted hours to get your perfect body? Now imagine if you could avoid those hours and hours of finding information for a successful recipe of how to get a dream body. If you have all that you need in one place, it would be a big fat tick in a box and value for your money. That would be a win!

In this book, I will explain what I mean by a magic pill. As I said, keep an open mind. If you make up your mind to believe in what you want and what you need, you can be unstoppable. I mean, with this pill's effects, you can achieve whatever you want. You can use the same directions for any of your dreams. This magic pill made my dreams come true, and I'm now chasing new ones. But it's important to have the right pill for you to achieve your dreams.

To get to the point where you have your perfect body, drive will play a crucial role. To be driven, you will need a pretty strong pill. For some people, one strong pill will be enough, but most people will need more than one strong pill to work effectively.

First, you will need an appointment with your doctor, the most qualified person to know what you require. To get the description of the pill, the doctor will first need to know a few things: what pill you need, how strong it should be, and how many. Second, he needs to know all about your problem. It's a proven fact, through the century as a standard process, that when you have a health issue, you go and see a doctor. You tell him all about your issue and desired outcome, and based on that, he can prescribe the right pills for you. It's always handy to be prepared before you see your doctor. You want to make sure to be clear on your issue, clear on your end result, be specific, and get everything in good detail. Remember, a doctor is a smart person who will focus on curing one problem at a time. Just like how you, as a smart person, will focus on solving one problem at a time. The basic process of solving problems is to break them down. Solving many problems at the same time can be too stressful, too confusing, and make it easy to lose track and control. It's just a fact.

The doctor prescribes the right pill. Happy days! All actions are in place, you go to the pharmacy, and get these magic pills, but wait, this magical pill looks different from what you imagined… but who cares, pills come in unusual colours and shapes, so with an open mind, you go for it. After a long journey home, you think about the future, full of excitement about how everything will look after taking these magic pills, seeing yourself successful with your perfect body. Once home, you stand in your kitchen, ready for changes. And the only thing on your mind is this one phrase, "Let's do it!".

You get the glass, fill it with water, and swallow the pill. Since it's different from a normal pill, it's hard to swallow. What do people do if something is hard or unusual? They quit! But you are not like all people! You know this magic pill will help, so a bit of difficulty will not stop you. Always keep in mind that you must believe in yourself. Your mind needs an explanation of what benefits you will receive from swallowing that magic pill. When all benefits are on the table, make a deal with the devil: your brain. The deal is to get the magic down and keep it inside. Remember, you must, time by time, conform; you still want this goal to keep your mind's trust in you and for the pill to do magic.

People often underestimate what they can achieve and how powerful it is when they believe. Ask this one question to yourself: What's the worst thing that can happen if you believe in yourself? And yes, there are always other people in whose eyes you will look stupid with your goals. Right now, help yourself and get this one phrase in your head: Who cares what they think! The quicker you understand that, the easier things will happen. Remember, you are doing something that they are too lazy or arrogant to do. You are already better than them!

It's difficult to swallow that pill when people comment or criticise you. And they will! There will be comments on your every step like, "How are you holding the glass", "Your glass is in the wrong hand", "The glass should be full of water because it's how all people prepare a glass before having a pill", or "Are you sure you need this much hassle to swallow this pill?". Comments are very annoying, but when people start to criticise, it is even worse, especially from people who are not the best example or people who have never been where you want to be. It's important to ignore comments and criticism from people who are not a great example in their own lives. There's nothing you can gain from them.

Tip for personal growth: "Keep people around you who lift you up, not drag you down".

What I mean by this is to keep people close to you who are positive, who are happy with your ideas and your achievements. People who support you and naturally push you up for a better and brighter life. They will motivate you naturally with their actions, achievements and their behaviours.

Try to avoid people around you who have a negative unconscious influence. These individuals are often unaware that they are stuck in negativity and inadvertently bring others down. It's in human nature to pay attention to criticism and comments from others; as a result, you might find yourself unable to reach your ideal body goal or succeed, simply because other people's opinions about you matter more than your own. I'm not suggesting that you should lock yourself away to escape all negativity, but rather that you should try to be around positive and motivated people to support your success. Ignoring negative comments is often the best way to handle them.

Comments from people who are loved or highly respected in your eyes should be treated differently. Usually, those comments are the most important to you. To deal with and effectively use those comments, your mind will need a mechanism to convert comments into action. Your mechanism should be, if someone tells you, "You can't do it!", this is the moment when you convert a demotivating phrase into driven action. You will do everything to prove that you can! You will prove you can be better; you will prove you keep your word. You can and will do it. All obstacles convert into driving actions. This magic pill, as like all pills that work, has potential side effects, and you should be prepared for that. Unfortunately, if you are not prepared, it is easy to destroy these magic pills and their effects. Don't worry, by the end of this book, you will be prepared enough to achieve your dreams and not lose your drive.

If your life is a mess, you can forget about magical pills doing wonders. Even a doctor would agree you can't live in a cold and damp property and at the same time expect to get rid of a feverish temperature with pills. So, for a magic pill to work, you must sort out your life first and start with basic things. Your finances, job, relationships, kids, and stress. To sort your life, you don't need to earn millions, have a very posh work title, or be in some kind of relationship just to be in one. Kids, if you have them, great, just make sure they have all the love and attention from you. If you don't have kids, even better, you can be more selfish and spend more time on yourself. You will see that your stress will go away when your life stabilises.

Don't try to sort everything in one go – tackle one thing at a time! You will start to see a chain reaction in your life as things start getting better, and your stress decreases. When your stress level is low, you will get bored with being too comfortable. Your life will be too stress-free. It's a nice feeling to have, but not for long. For you, as an ambitious person, you will need the next big thing to start happening in your life, and that's the moment for you to go and get that magic pill and swallow it.

A pill is naturally designed to perform at its best performance but only if it is strong enough or you take enough of them. For different people with different needs, one person's pill might need to be strong, while another person will need more than one pill to do magic. I need to warn you! You probably will get addicted to this magic pill. After seeing the amazing results, you will be in a trap for the greater future, as you will want them over and over for several reasons.

Let me tell you something surprising: everyone knows what this special magic pill is! So, let's dive in, and I'll explain in each chapter what is what, just bear with me.

Are you the right person for the Magic Pill?

The magic pill is not for everyone! After reading this book, you might realise that this magic pill isn't for you, and that's perfectly okay. It's crucial to understand what is on your priority list. Your mindset and your priorities must align for magic to happen. Everyone has their own priorities, and what matters to one person may not matter to another. Don't waste your time on things that aren't important to you.

Let's say you might think about losing weight and having a beach body because it's trendy and everyone is doing it before summer. You enjoy the idea of being active and looking good on hot summer days, especially when wearing minimal clothing. However, if it's just an idea and not your new lifestyle, it won't become your main priority. Years of habits will take over your new ideas.

Habits are one thing that can hold you back from being the right person for magic pills, but let's look into how diet and physical activity choices play into this. For instance, your long-standing eating habits, such as enjoying decent-sized portions and snacking between meals, will overpower your desire to lose weight. Weakness will always win, and you'll get nowhere. The same applies to physical activity. You might like the idea of being active, but often other things seem more important. Realising how beneficial it can be to have at least one good hour of exercise and how it can positively impact your physical and mental health would make you rethink your actions. People need to be active for their bodies to work better, but we often find more and more excuses to avoid activities.

A very common excuse for avoiding exercise is a tough day at work, when your boss is in a bad mood, and everything seems to go wrong. It's one of those days where whatever you do, it feels like nothing works. And often, you don't even realise that these days happen more often than you'd like. So, what if you're not in the mood for physical activity? You may feel drained and powerless, and this becomes a reason to simply go home and relax on your comfortable sofa in front of the TV. I've been there, felt that, and made countless excuses to stay in that comfort zone because it was my priority at the time. However, what people often don't realise is that after a difficult day at work, the best thing you can do is engage in some physical activity. I understand how difficult it is to decide whether to stay in your comfort zone or push yourself to exercise. Let me tell you, without your magic pill, you'll often choose your sofa and TV to end the day. That's the raw truth we must face.

I always stand for a physically good and healthy body, and it should be near the top of your priority list. But while it's not your top priority, don't waste your time with other ideas. Ideas are great to have, but you need commitment because whatever you do, without commitment, you will fail. This occurs simply because old habits will take over, and you will eventually come out feeling even worse than before. The point is, you must understand where your priorities stand.

This book could be exactly what you need. Because you are reading this book means you are the right person for a magic pill dose. It is a fact that if you are reading a book about achieving your perfect body, inside you, you have ambition, and this ambition just needs magic for greater success. Now, look at yourself from the side. This book in your hands, what does it say about you? It tells a remarkable story! The beginning of your new life and your new lifestyle. With this book in your hands, you are the person who wants a bit more from life, and you are ready to do something about it, but the confusion that nothing works to achieve your perfect body leads you back to disappointment. Can you remember all those countless times when you probably didn't even get halfway through your perfect body goal, but found yourself back where you were before you started? Whatever you do, you fail over and over, and as a result, your motivation is destroyed. After failure, it's so difficult to find the courage to start again. The thought of how this perfect body goal just goes in circles and gets nowhere will drain you out. At the same time, ask yourself: how do you manage other things in life, and how have other life goals been achieved? For other goals, you always had magic pills, but you never realised. This time, it will be different. This time, you will be aware of it, and being aware will help you to focus on the right things.

So, let me answer this chapter's question. Are you the right person for The Magic Pill? And the answer is one hundred percent, YES! You deserve to live better, feel better, and look better.

Be aware!

A few main characteristics can influence the realisation of dreams. You must be aware that these factors can prevent most people from living differently and in a better way. Let's examine each obstacle more closely.

The first obstacle will be people being foolish. You can be foolish with your decisions and attitude, but eventually, this will lead to failure and prevent you from achieving your goals. Being foolish means you are not learning from mistakes. This is a common problem for most people. I'll explain similarities in two examples: relationships and the goal to achieve your dream body. For example, many people find themselves stuck in toxic relationships and cannot break free from this cycle. They don't see an opportunity to escape at the right time and, as a result, they jump from one poor relationship to another, repeating the same mistakes and experiencing the same outcomes. The main reason for this is that, for these people, this lifestyle is the norm. They don't even realise that there are different ways to live. When you are in that mindset, it will lead you to avoid crucial steps. One step to escape this cycle includes: "learn from previous experiences and mistakes".

You could be one of the lucky ones and have someone next to you to point out what you could do differently or better to step out of this locked circle. You need to understand that if there is someone whose lifestyle is something that you would like, and this person is happy to help you with good advice from their experiences, don't be foolish, listen and see beyond yourself. Learn from mistakes and discover that there are different relationships possible, those that are full of care and full of love. Imagine living a different kind of standard life, a much better life with balance, harmony, and happiness with an incredible, love-filled relationship!

If you look back on all those many times when you worked hard on your dream body, you will see the same pattern. Your perfect body journeys will have the same locked circle, similar to the unhealthy relationship example. I'm not pointing out that you have a toxic relationship, not at all; you could be in the best relationship you could imagine, but for the locked circle example, I compare poor relationships with poor success in improving your body. Around you, you probably have someone with poor relationships which never really seem to get better because they never analyse and never learn from mistakes. Do it differently this time. Understand how important it is to stop and look back on your mistakes, analyse them and take good things that worked and avoid things that didn't work. I want you to be better and smarter this time, but before you do that, look at yourself from a different perspective again and recognise how you have become stuck in this cycle due to these repeated mistakes. This observed side information will help you to address them.

Ask yourself the question. Did you ever analyse earlier failures? Start with a question. What didn't work well the last time you tried to improve your body? For example, get into detail about your diet. If you have been in this locked circle, it's a fact that you couldn't come up with the best diet to fit you and your lifestyle – one that shows remarkable results and, at the same time, can be sustainable further in your future. Nowadays, when everything has been made "quick and easy to get", people's nature is lazier and more laid back as a result, which often takes over patient and challenging work. In the twenty-first century, more people like to skip important information and good, in-depth research, which could have led them to different kinds of successes. Let's take an example in the perfect body journey, starting from the part where a person wants to put effort into losing weight. It usually starts with finding an idea of what will be the best and fastest way to lose weight, and because of the overwhelming access to information nowadays, people often choose to get inspirational ideas in some quick and effortless ways. Instead of spending hours reading or watching good research on how to lose weight, people will choose to get ideas from "trusted sources". This involves the people around you, such as your friends and family, or work colleagues. people who have lately had a remarkable body makeover in their weight loss. It's amazing to know a person who lost a good proportion of weight and looks good at this moment, but people quite often forget two things that could be very misleading.

Your "trusted sources" may not always be the best example for you, simply because there is a saying, "What works for one may not work for another", and this saying exists for a reason. This one method that works perfectly for your friend in his journey to lose weight can be perfect for him and his lifestyle, but not for you and your lifestyle. For example, a friend with an improved body and impressive results on losing weight started something new and is extremely impressed with this strange, crazy diet, "the cucumber diet". Cucumbers, as vegetables, are one of the best products to consume to lose weight because they are low in calories. Cucumbers are made up of around 96 percent water, which is great food to keep you on a low-calorie diet and, at the same time, fills you up. So, without any research, you take advice from a trusted source, your friend (the person whom you have known for many years and know would never lie to you), and jump straight into this super cucumber diet that has produced amazing results, just because it works very well for your friend. Let's stop here and ask two questions to ourselves.

1. Is my lifestyle (food-wise) exactly the same as my friend's lifestyle?
2. Do I commit now to forever live on cucumbers?

The answers to both questions will be available in a split second because every person has unique needs and wishes when it comes to food. Your food lifestyle, for sure, will be different and unique when you start to compare it with your friend's food lifestyle. For example, a friend can be a vegetarian, but you are a proper meat-eater. The friend's mindset is all about vegetables, but yours is not. It's easy for him to use cucumber as the main product in his diet, so it will be sustainable, and he can live the rest of his life adding cucumbers to his normal diet without any issues, but you love your meat, and are you ready to give up your meat dishes for cucumbers? Probably not, because it's not your sustainable food lifestyle, and therefore, there will not be a commitment to live on cucumber for the rest of your life.

A common mistake people make when choosing their diet is selecting one that isn't sustainable or suited to their lifestyle. These poorly chosen diets may work for a short period, but soon you'll find yourself back at the starting point because the diet wasn't right for you and couldn't be maintained. Many popular diets are believed to help with weight loss, but if they aren't sustainable for your future life, they can trap you in a cycle of repeated attempts and failure.

Another mistake occurs when people see impressive results from trusted sources, but these results are only recent. Usually, it's enough to take that diet as a perfect example and give yourself the green light to start a weight loss journey with an unusual diet. By recent, I mean these impressive weight-loss results are just initial, quick outcomes. If someone is overweight, nearly every new diet will show impressive results in a short period, provided they strictly follow the diet. These first impressive results happen because the body isn't scared to lose extra fat. Our bodies are remarkable; overweight bodies on new lifestyle changes will adapt and respond accordingly. If the body loses a good portion of fat, it still has plenty of reserves and will stay calm without panic to survive. Your trusted source's recent results can be very misleading. Results from someone who has been on a weight loss journey for a long time – meaning at least a year – would be a more reliable example for you to consider, helping you research how it might fit into your lifestyle.

Be aware that people are easily influenced by those who are not fit and not looking after themselves, but those people always have a strong opinion on what's good and what's wrong. Individuals who neglect themselves and those around them can be dangerous to someone like you who has a brighter vision for the future. They often believe they know what is best for you, and even if they don't, they tend to be very convincing in their comments about you. Somehow, they seem to have a gift for strong criticism, and a simple comment like, "don't be stupid," "it's not for you," or "why are you torturing yourself?" can quickly turn your mindset around and cause you to lose all motivation and excitement for this new chapter in your life. All mistakes, caused by negative comments from others, self-doubt, and being stuck in a loop are common problems that can hinder people from achieving their dream of a perfect body. However, the main issue is that the only thing missing is this 'magical pill' for success in your journey towards the perfect body. You can always start by analysing yourself, identifying what didn't work and what did, which will allow you to understand and correct your course. Remember, to understand what works well is just as important as what doesn't.

The second obstacle, why people hold themselves back from achieving their dreams, is their laziness. 'Lazy' is a strong word, and usually, people become quickly upset if someone calls them lazy. Years ago, I used to get upset when someone I cared about called me lazy because I always viewed myself as a hard-working person. Over time, I learnt to accept my lazy side. Now, I am truly honest with myself and can admit that I can be lazy about trivial things in my life. Simple tasks like repainting walls or reorganising the loft, which I have planned to do for a year but find unimportant enough not to do, fall into this category. I might be lazy about homework and chores around the house, but instead, I go to the gym, push myself, or spend hours with my lovely wife on long walks. For important aspects of my life, such as self-improvement, work, relationships, family, commitments, and promises, laziness is not an option. There, I refuse to be lazy because these are the things that ensure a brighter future for my family and me.

In the past few years, I observed people around me and came to the conclusion that I would say a small number of people are more laid back in their lives by nature, but all the others are busy trying to achieve more from life. Look around yourself, at family, friends, or colleagues at work, to get your own picture of who is busy and who is laid back, and try to see which category you fit into. If you think you could be one of those laid-back people but want to change it, you need to find a purpose in life. After reading this book, you will have the opportunity to have this magical pill to change your life from laid back to productively busy, and you will be busy for the right reasons.

So, how about all these other, remarkably busy people? For a person to feel and appear busy daily, it is easy for him to believe he is highly productive. Moreover, positive comments from those around him, often those complimenting him about his lifestyle, serve as solid evidence of someone with no spare time at all. It seems impossible that this person harbours even a hint of laziness, but if you are so active, busy, and productive, then why can't you make your dreams come true? Being busy, active, and productive in life, yet still failing in realising your dreams? The answer is simple: it is because, in most cases, people are productive and busy focusing on various things, but somehow avoid and neglect their focus on achieving their true goals.

Let's look at a remarkably busy person from the side. Now, in your mind, look around and find a person; it could be in your family, a close friend, or a work colleague. It's easier to imagine if it's a person you see and know daily, but choose the remarkably busy person, and like us all, I can guarantee this person will have some dreams and wishes for a better life. You can see and understand from daily conversations with this person how active he or she is; it even looks like this person never stops. This person has a strict routine, work, and daily tasks like picking up kids from school, cooking, taking kids to their activities, shopping, washing, and on weekends, they're fully into gardening, cleaning, and ironing. This person clearly doesn't stop, and yet dreams stay only dreams for this person. Often in conversation with this "not a lazy person", you can hear wishes about how great it would be to lose weight, get stronger, be successful, or be healthier, but it never happens. It just proves that laziness or being busy is not a problem, but it's focused on different priorities. Still, we need to understand that we can't escape from daily tasks, because they are an essential part of our lives.

Then, how do we achieve our dreams? To achieve your dreams, you will need to be a bit selfish and find some time for yourself. To free up time, you will need to prioritise what's important and what you can sacrifice. Those can be unimportant things or habits, like going shopping three times a week instead of planning and doing it once a week. Maybe ironing bedding isn't that important! What could be the worst thing that happens if you decide not to iron your bedding? Instead, use this time to invest in yourself, for example, in physical activity or in doing some research on how to improve yourself. I'll tell you what the worst thing that can happen is; your partner can be a bit grumpy with uneven bedding, but your partner can't argue with you about skipping ironing and investing time in your health and body!

Let's look at another sacrifice you can make. For example, your garden is the best-looking garden on your street. All those hours that have been spent every weekend looking after every flower and every corner of the garden have finally paid off. Your garden looks wonderful, and you have been busy keeping it like that for years. At the same time, you always dreamed of having a perfect body. You would like to look and feel good, but all those hours spent gardening, half-bending on your knees, leave you stiff and tired, stopping you from wanting to do any extra physical exercise and from having a dream body. It's a split feeling; you are happy about your wonderful-looking garden, but physically, you feel drained.

So, how about trading your lovely garden for a wonderful-looking you? Let's consider where the greater benefits lie. Spending time in the garden and having others admire your effort, or focusing on yourself, doing research and physical activities for a healthier life, where people will notice how good and healthy you look and feel? Make yourself the priority, but keep your garden simple and easy to maintain, as simple as an hour a week to mow the lawn. This way, you can free up your entire weekend for activities that will help you improve yourself. Focus on what truly matters and shift your focus to the right things; they should help your dreams come true.

If your focus is on the wrong things, there will be consequences. Unfortunately, you will experience extra difficulty in your life. That's not a feeling you want! Feeling what many people know as: "I can't be bothered"? We all know this sentence, and when we have this moment with this phrase, we kind of know that nothing good will happen. This feeling is the first step to laziness. You will automatically start to skip and avoid things that can lead you to consequences, and these consequences will lead you to a poor habit. A habit of acting lazily. By admitting and making clear which daily activities you have been lazy about and why, you could help yourself in your progress to make your dreams come true. People often try to avoid things that are outside their comfort zone. Normally, three things cause laziness: "unknown", "never done" and "hard to do".

First, consider the "unknown things". If you don't understand how your body responds and works during potential changes or don't know where to start on your journey to a perfect body, it can become intimidating. This may lead you to think, "I can't be bothered to do this." A combination of the unknown and an attitude like 'I can't be bothered' can cause someone to become lazy, and all these factors may result in stopping the pursuit of their dreams. Instead, treat the unknown changes as known ones. Put some effort into doing at least a little research on where to begin, what the main steps are, and what to expect, so it doesn't feel like an unachievable journey. With that understanding, you won't develop the attitude, "I can't be bothered."

Second, "never done". How about things you've never done before? Completely change your diet, join the gym, or start being active, things that have never been part of your life. People naturally tend to avoid new things and change because they don't like them. However, for changes to work well, you should like and love them, and they should fit your lifestyle. If you like this new, completely changed diet and enjoy every bite, even missing this new taste between meals, you will start to love the idea. The same applies to becoming active. Find an activity that fits into your lifestyle, and make sure it makes you feel good and comfortable. If you love this new idea and can easily adopt it without stressing about how, when, or if you have time for these changes, then recent changes in your life will not seem like a big deal and will be easier to overcome. To avoid laziness towards things you've never done, make sure, before starting something entirely new, to consider if it suits your lifestyle, and try it out to see if you like what you eat or do.

Third, "hard to do". People often start a new chapter in their lives, but when it begins to get tough or obstacles appear, they tend to quit because it's usually the easiest choice. When it becomes hard, you shouldn't stop; instead, aim for more challenging paths. Hard isn't always that bad; we often exaggerate how difficult it is. Pause and ask yourself, "Is it truly hard or just a bit difficult?" or "Did I just make it seem that way?" Most likely, you'll realise it's not as bad as it looks. This mindset helps you continue pursuing your dream goals and leaves laziness behind. Sometimes, you hope for magic to happen, and now you can have this magic pill along with extra support. This magic pill contains all the ingredients to help you overcome laziness and achieve your perfect body dream. With this magic pill, you will be able to overcome all obstacles on your journey to achieving the perfect body.

The next obstacle is quitting. Many people give up when things get tough, lack patience because it's too long, or they, by nature, start something and never finish, quitting midway. To achieve this dream, quitting is not even an option. If you find yourself in the past starting things and never finishing them, you could potentially find a block preventing you from reaching your end goal. That doesn't mean you shouldn't try to achieve your dreams. It's important to admit and acknowledge this. What is the normal reason why people tend to quit? As I often mention, the main reason to quit is when things start to get hard, and when it's hard, you have the option to step away from whatever you do. The same applies if the journey is too long; it can start to become boring. When there's no action in your journey, people lose interest and excitement about the end goal. It's like running a marathon without a magic pill. At the beginning, it's exciting, and you're full of motivation, then halfway through, it starts to get hard, and there's still so much to run. Then it begins to get a bit boring because nothing is changing, and you don't see the finish line. The next potential step will be to quit. So, when you have that urge to quit, stop and use your 'magic pill' to overcome it.

The confidence obstacle is that people with high confidence levels or overconfidence can create reasons for not reaching their dream goals because, thinking highly of themselves, they build an invisible wall. This wall prevents them from taking in more information when they feel strong and smart in certain areas of their life. It's their choice! Each of us possesses a certain level of confidence in some aspects of life. However, a small dose of confidence can motivate us to achieve our dreams. When kept in moderation, confidence can be positive; for example, a little self-confidence can be a boost. As you know, confidence can lead to success and help overcome many obstacles in life. It can encourage someone to take risks or pursue goals, but without confidence, others might avoid opportunities due to self-doubt. Confidence helps build a strong, powerful personality; it gives you the courage to make decisions, believe in yourself, and recover from mistakes even stronger and smarter. So, if you have a good level of confidence and little self-doubt, you're more likely to achieve your dreams and goals. A boost of confidence in high-pressure environments like competitive sports, business, or leadership plays a vital role in success. However, I am talking about just enough confidence, not confidence that makes a person act as if they know everything. If someone acts as if they are always right and disrespects others, that is overconfidence, which can be viewed negatively. Overconfidence is often seen negatively because it is associated with dismissiveness and a lack of respect for others. These traits can prevent people from reaching remarkable success.

To succeed in this journey toward achieving the perfect body, you must open your mind and accept that you don't know everything. Be willing to learn and give this magic pill a try. Most people, by nature, may believe they know better how to attain the perfect body, yet they still fail to reach their dreams and goals. As you are putting so much effort into reading this book, do yourself a favour. Be kind to yourself, make this journey as easy as possible, and let go of thoughts like "I know better how to get my perfect body." Don't block your path to success. Be a bigger person, overcome your overconfidence, and give this magic pill a try for your success. This magic pill helped me achieve my ideal body goal, and from there, I continued to succeed in all other areas of my life. Don't do this for me or anyone else. Do it for yourself.

The last and very strong obstacle that often doesn't allow people to be successful is their comfort zone. All the things that prevent you from achieving more are consequences of staying in your comfort zone. Let's examine how a person behaves and feels when in a comfortable state and what consequences they may face. So, what is comfort? The comfort zone is that mental and physical space where we feel at our best and safest because there are no surprises or demands beyond our usual capacity. However, if we remain within these boundaries for too long, we might become reluctant to try new things, even when those things could bring about positive change.

A mental comfort zone, for example, is when a person feels at ease in their current job, avoiding new challenges like a promotion or extra responsibilities to remain in a safe and stress-free environment. And why not? You have work, you know how to do it, everything goes according to plan, and there's no stress because there are no additional responsibilities. It sounds like a dream job; that's what you call a comfort zone. While this stability exists, the person happily avoids any upcoming opportunities to grow and improve in their workplace or through self-development. So, in one word, they are "stuck". When stuck in this comfort zone, it can feel like the sweet spot. Over time, there arises a feeling of wanting to change something because the job becomes boring as you do the same tasks repeatedly. However, this feeling is often suppressed by the stronger feeling of stressless comfort. This is the moment when a person rethinks their job! Now, imagine yourself in this person's position. Reflect on a time when you felt comfortable with your lifestyle. You avoided extra activities because you felt healthy and fit, discovering takeaway foods to save time and reduce the pressure of cooking. This comfort zone fosters a relaxing lifestyle, no stress about cooking in the evenings, just relaxing in front of the TV with a takeaway in hand. It's your safe place and routine, knowing where to order food and what to watch. Gradually, you start avoiding doing other things like going for walks, seeing friends, or tackling basic chores around the house. And now, you find yourself stuck! But you begin to feel uncomfortable with your body and lifestyle. Yet, your stronger, safer feeling continues to dominate. At that moment, you realise you're beginning to feel unhappy with yourself, but at the same time, your comfort zone takes over your life. You remain stuck, unhappy, and unable to make a change.

Physical comfort zones can lead to similar outcomes. For example, choosing rest over exercise may feel more comfortable initially, but over time, it can negatively affect health and vitality. Without physical activity, you will notice consequences, such as your body feeling stiff and painful. Gradually, every movement begins to feel uncomfortable. For instance, when standing up from the sofa, you might feel a sharp pain in your lower back, signalling to your brain: "Hey, take it slowly!" That sensation causes you to slow down and can make you look unfit. What about your knees? After sitting on the sofa for hours, you're sure to notice that those first steps are awkward. The longer your legs stay bent, the more that uncomfortable, sometimes painful feeling in your joints makes you feel old. Are these familiar feelings? The problem arises when you become aware of them, but your comfort zone prevents you from staying active. Both mental and physical comfort zones tend to be stronger because it's natural to feel safe. Usually, people only step out of these zones when something significant happens in their lives. Usually, something negative occurs, prompting people to try to save what they can. Too often, it's already too late. However, it's not too late to leave your comfort zone; what's more concerning is the damage already done by being overweight, joint pain from daily movements, and the pain of sitting in one position for long periods, as your back starts aching. Then, there's a wake-up call, and suddenly everyone tries to catch up with time to address health issues. As you age, you realise that your health is the most important thing to look after. Remember, the human body is built for exercise and movement, and if you allow your body to stop, you'll find it difficult to recover. The comfort zone can be a place of rest, but it shouldn't become a long-term destination. Push yourself beyond your comfort zone for real magic to occur.

Throughout your life, you probably follow only one standard way of living without realising there are other options. Keep an open mind, analyse yourself, and make some changes to improve your life. It's time for you to discover a better and more fulfilling life. With this magic pill, you will break free from this locked circle and succeed in any way you desire.

Me and pill

I discovered this pill, and it worked very well for me. I'm an average person who has gone through and am still going through the journey for the perfect body, because it really never ends. I had my magic pill, and it worked a miracle, but now I need to admit I'm officially addicted to this pill. For any of my new dreams or goals, I have this one strong magic pill, or sometimes I need more than one pill, depending on the situation. It all started when my wife and I decided to improve our already good relationship, I mean, an incredibly good relationship. You would ask: Why improve something already great? We are all constantly changing, so some of the things that were great yesterday may not be great today. I don't mean to say that we change overnight; it usually happens over a longer period. To be in a great relationship, you must put effort into it. I have a wonderful wife, the best son I could wish for, a job that I love to do, good family finances and no stress. My life was sorted. It was a perfect time for the magic pill.

So, going back to the beginning, my wife changed her lifestyle many years ago, and since then, she has always championed a healthy lifestyle and a fit body. Being in this relationship, I naturally adopted a healthier lifestyle as well, but it didn't significantly improve my appearance. I mean, I wasn't expecting a massive bodybuilding physique, but I wanted a nice, healthy, well-defined body with clear muscles on display. So, I decided that one of the things I would focus on was "I'll improve my body so I can take my shirt off at any moment and feel good about how I look." And as a cherry on top, I was hoping that my wife would appreciate my new look. It might sound silly, but sometimes silly things can make a big difference. And for me, a happy wife means a happy life!

I'm a family person, working eight hours, five days a week. I'm not one of those perfect muscle-looking influencers who live in the gym. Not even one of those who can work and improve their body every single day and look awesome every single moment. It's just their lifestyle, and I'm probably a bit jealous, but I'm like most of you: family is my whole world. This is a normal standard lifestyle for most people. If you are single, that's good too. Invest and concentrate time on yourself. If you have a family, it's brilliant. Your priorities should be all around your loved ones. In these circumstances, this magical pill is very needed and very handy to have.

That's me, a family person with daily routine tasks. Job, home shopping, and taking my son to training. Sounds familiar? Sounds like your busy life? But is it? Lots of people find excuses not to have time. The most common sentence I hear from people who say they want to start something new is "I don't have time." You have time. You need to want it and make it. Sitting in front of the TV, I thought I was such a busy person, and I deserved this moment with my favourite TV show. And yes, I deserve it, but once or twice a week, not every evening. So, because I had my pill and I wanted to start gym sessions, I was driven to make time for myself. My wonderful wife and I scheduled weekdays, who's doing what and on which day. We created this schedule to work around all of us, plus I had my time, and she had hers. Even then, in the evening, we still found an hour to spend with each other.

On top of my busy week, I started drafting this book, and I needed to find time for my closed, isolated moment a day to put some words down and not be disturbed by anyone. For that, I needed peace and quiet, me time. That was the moment when my addiction to magic pills, again, was very handy. It's amazing how this pill can drive you to make things happen. So, I found some extra me time. I decided to wake up every morning at four o'clock and spend one hour writing before work. Why on earth would you wake up at four o'clock to draft a book? I had this pill and the magic with it, and because of that, I couldn't see a problem with freeing up some time early in the mornings.

Let's get back to the perfect body journey. Thanks to magical pills, I changed my diet, and I lost a good portion of weight. I have had an incredible change in my body physically and visually. With losing weight, I could start to see my muscles popping out on my body, and let me tell you, it was a nice feeling when I began to see results. One day after my gym session, I caught myself looking in the mirror and admiring what I had achieved so far. Time by time, out of curiosity, I check my Weight App to see how I have changed or progressed since I started this perfect body journey. In the app, including the weight check, I have sixteen different parameters, plus other options like comparing days and months to see which direction you are moving. So, I went through all the parameters, and I compared them, before and now. I probably did that to boost my confidence. It makes you feel better to see positive progress, but I realised that with losing fat, I lost muscle mass as well. So that was disappointing! I aimed to lose fat, not muscles. At that point in my journey, I didn't know that your body uses muscles as fuel if you are not looking after your protein intake to build muscles. Fat is more difficult to burn because it is the safety layer around your body. Then, I was back to researching how it works and what to change, but all the changes led back to the kitchen. Now it's started to be more challenging. I needed to reframe my diet. In my new diet, I made sure I had my focus on the correct protein amount for my gym days and the correct amount for rest days, and still at the same time, I should be in a calorie deficit. The challenge was accepted, and I was back on track to lose fat and grow muscle.

To have the magic pill and see the results of it, I looked back into the past, and I realised I had this magic pill addiction before. I had a strong pill to help with quitting smoking. And it did magic then. I quit smoking. It was more than ten years ago. And after all these years, I'm back on pills to achieve my new big goal, my perfect body.

In this chapter, I just wanted to show you that I'm one of you and I have been where you are now. I made my own mistakes only because I didn't have this magical pill at that time. I had and still have my journey with a busy family life. However, I changed my lifestyle with the help of "The Magic Pill". Now, I feel like I have multiple successes in my life, so I hope to share some of the examples of my successful journey that would allow you to trust me and try this Magic Pill to fix your problems.

The Magic Pill

In this chapter, you will discover where to find the magic pill and how strong the pill should be for it to work effectively. And perhaps, it will not be enough with just one strong pill; you might need more than one to keep you driving further towards success. Finally, you will learn what this magical pill actually is.

It all begins with where to obtain this magic pill. So, where would you usually go, and who do you typically see if you need a pill? I can confidently say that your answer would be a doctor. The first step would usually be to make an appointment with your doctor, who knows best what pill you need. The good news is, you are not actually ill! Yes, you have a problem, but it's not a medical illness. So, if you are not ill, how can you get pills without a doctor's help? Here's some good news: you don't need to waste your time, nerves, or sit in queues stressing about what the doctor will say, because for this magic pill, you don't need a doctor. You can also avoid awkward conversations with strangers about personal problems. All you need is yourself, as someone who knows what's best for you. Still, you should find some time for yourself to make an appointment, as it's part of the process for the magic pill to work. Find a peaceful and comfortable place away from daily routines, such as treating yourself to a drink at your local café. Set aside an hour to plan how to get that magic pill and make it as effective as possible.

Do exercise. Think about your achievements. Choose one of the things that you are proudest of the most. Now dig into your past. What was the trigger and reason for you to achieve that achievement?

Now, when you find the reason, be honest with yourself. The reason can be nice, stupid, or ugly, but it's your reason. Remember, it was good enough to drive you to achieve your goal. So, apply this method to drive you to your perfect body goal. As you probably understand, this magic pill will not look like all pills. This magic pill is what I call: **"The best reason is the one worth dying for"**. To achieve goals, you always have the best reason behind them.

Many years ago, someone close to me said: "You will always work hard in your life". It wasn't meant in a bad way, but rather as a fact. This was based on the fact that I am a shy and quiet person. To this person, I always looked like the typical unconfident teenager. You can probably imagine that one kid among friends who always considers consequences before acting. That kid is the opposite of all his friends. Back then, I was more of a follower who tried to please everyone and avoid standing up for my own opinions. That phrase about needing to work hard all my life stuck in my mind for years. I was only a teenager then, and my view of life wasn't to work hard forever. I envisioned myself working in an office, dressed smartly and being a respectful person like my father. Only a few years ago, I realised I had been unconsciously doing everything to prove I could be more and that I wouldn't be forced to work hard all my life. In my career, I took on all challenges and opportunities to be more than just a shy, head-down person. I accepted challenges and had a magical drive for self-growth and self-development. But all of this comes from somewhere, and that somewhere was a trigger from my past. This comment, about me "working hard all my life," was the real reason my mind naturally shifted and created what I call a magical pill. My magic pill became a reason to prove that person wrong about me. For some, this reason might sound silly, but for my mind, it created the strongest motivation to keep going. I am grateful for this trigger and reason from my past.

The secret to success is having a magic pill, "your best reason." Your journey usually begins with one strong reason, but is this reason strong enough to be a magic pill? Let's explore a few scenarios with the magic pill being weak, not good enough to overcome obstacles, and strong enough to be unstoppable. The first scenario involves a weak magic pill. In a world where friends, colleagues, and everyone in the media talk about being healthy and fit, this is the latest modern trend. You decide not to be a black sheep but to join the modern crowd and follow the trend.

In the end, this modern approach seems like the right thing to do. It's all about being healthy and fit. So, in your mind, you have a perfect reason, and because of that, it sounds like you have your magic pill as well. I'll tell you right now, it will never work. You don't have a clear goal. How will you know when you are truly healthy and fit? Where will your finish line be? Any moment could be enough for you to stop. You will fail because you don't know what the end goal looks like. What benefits will you gain from being modern? This will never be a sufficient reason because you love your habits, enjoy living comfortably, and have always loved tasty food. These factors will overpower you very quickly. It will be difficult to restrain yourself. Ultimately, we only live once! That will be the best excuse to give up. If that excuse works, then your magic pill wasn't strong enough.

However, for the second scenario, I'll provide three compelling examples that use the magic pill. In the first scenario, you will be a fortunate person. You have been approached by an agent from the world's most popular magazine. This agent is seeking a natural, good-looking person for next year's January issue cover story under the theme "New Modern, Healthy, and Lean." You are offered a once-in-a-lifetime contract to sign. The contract states you will feature on the cover of the world's most popular magazine and receive a generous half a million pounds in pay. It sounds very impressive to be famous and to have half a million pounds in your pocket. As always, there are rules. Men must attain a lean fourteen percent body fat, and women a lean twenty percent for the photo shoot. Is that a good enough reason for you to endure hardship? I am entirely confident it would serve as a bulletproof reason for those seeking more from life. In this case, you have a clear goal: reach a fourteen percent body fat level by January. You know the target number on the scales, so you don't stop until you achieve it. The best part is the end goal: half a million pounds deposited into your bank account. This is your "best reason worth dying for," and it will motivate you to succeed.

The second strong pill scenario will be related to money only for a lot of people; money can be a priority and a main drive. You win a lottery. 168 million. But this lottery is designed to make people healthier, and there are rules to follow. You will have access to the first ten million only if you achieve a clear fitness goal. Your goal will be to achieve fifteen percent body fat, but if you want to keep getting access to the next ten million, you must sustain this lean body continuously at fifteen percent. Will that reason drive you to get to the first ten million, and will it keep driving you through the other months for more? I would sign up for that lottery. How about you?

Let's look at another perfect reason. Some people don't care about popularity or money, so the previous example wouldn't drive them to success because it is not their priority. Let's say your priorities sit with health, happiness, love, respect and a stressless lifestyle. Remember that everyone has different views and needs in their lives. It's important to understand and respect them. A very strong example in most cases is when it's nearly too late. People have the best reason to live after they have nearly lost their life. It's that moment in hospital when the doctor tells you must get fitter to be healthier and live. This is a magic pill. The only downside is that doctors don't tell you exactly what you need to achieve to stay healthy and have the opportunity to live your life, but in this case, people automatically have the magic pill for them to stay alive. All other values will just follow. There will be love and respect from close ones because this person fights for his life. This person will start feeling healthier and happier. A stressless lifestyle will take over because all decisions will be made to avoid stressful situations. I hope, with all my heart, that YOU will not wait for it to be too late to have a reason to change your life for the better.

To begin working on your ideal body, whether it involves losing weight, gaining weight, building muscle, or simply maintaining an already perfect physique, it always starts with your mind. As I mentioned earlier, your strong reason will set your mindset straight and help you achieve your goals. Remember, a strong and healthy mind will lead to a strong, healthy, and beautiful body! Some individuals associate having a "perfect" body with being healthy and physically fit. They believe that maintaining a specific body composition will contribute to overall well-being, reduce the risk of certain health conditions, and improve their quality of life. And they would be right! It is like a circle. A strong mind helps to attain a perfect body, and a perfect body helps keep a strong mind. It's a win-win, perfect body and strong mind!

You probably want to ask; how do I get to a strong and healthy mind? And the answer is, it starts only with you and your decisions. Only you can build this mindset. As I mentioned in the last paragraph, you must sort out your life at least to a level where you don't need to think or stress constantly about something. Let's say you've sorted things in your private life that didn't give you peace, and with that, you move away from the main stress. If you don't have this constant stress and life calms down, you will begin to get bored. That will be your sign that you are fully ready for a new challenge. But don't wait for that moment; if your mind is clear, it's time to act.

Do you have "the very best reason" that is worth dying for? Ask yourself that question before setting a goal for your perfect body. It all begins with questions I ask people when they tell me they want to lose weight and start their journey to a perfect body. The questions I ask are: Why? What is your reason? And is your reason strong enough to keep you going through tough times? Usually, the first answers are not the actual real best reasons. Only after some time, digging into the past and discovering your trigger, will you find the real reason. These are the very best reasons that can vary for different people. For example:

I want to prove to everyone that I'm more capable than they think.

I'll do whatever it takes to get attention from the person I like.

I'll do it because not everyone can, and that will make me special.

I want to transform my life and lifestyle, so I feel that I am someone special to someone.

I want to be better than anyone else I know.

I nearly died; I desperately want to live.

These are some of the reasons that can change your mindset. Most often, the best reasons are those where you desperately want to prove something to someone.

It always begins with one reason, which could be exceptionally strong, but over time, people usually add more reasons to strengthen their motivation–for example, me. My main and initial reason for pursuing my ideal body was to appear more attractive and more attractive to my wife, so she retains a little extra spark after all these years together. When a couple has been together for many years, they naturally lose some of that initial spark. With time and love, people start to believe that their partner will love them regardless of how they look. And it's true! Most people accept each other as they are and what their partner looks like. That's because they love and rely on each other to accept them no matter how they appear. Due to love and support from their partner, many stop trying to impress each other. Over time, this can become a problem, but no one talks about it to avoid hurting the partner's feelings. We all need to realise that relationships require maintenance and growth over the years. Sometimes, we don't notice or feel these changes, but both we and our relationships are always evolving. Don't make the mistake of taking your relationship for granted. Remember, a strong relationship depends on effort from both sides; you both need to actively work at making it stronger.

Back to my primary strong reason. It was time to change my lifestyle and reignite the spark in our relationship. I had my magic pill, my perfect method to reach my goal. The main reason was to become more attractive to my wife. By doing so, I also hoped to spark her sexual attraction towards me. It might sound embarrassing, silly, or even desperate, but that's not the point. The key was to have a very strong reason. No matter what that reason was, the important thing was to have a strong reason to achieve my goal. Even now, I stand by my opinion: if you can improve sexual attraction in a long-term relationship, you can't wish for more. It was my first super-strong, magical pill for the perfect body. My perfect reason for having the drive to achieve an excellent physical appearance.

After some time, when people noticed changes in my body, I received plenty of compliments, and my response was always pride that I was on a journey to achieve the perfect body. From this, I automatically created my next 'magic pill'. I'm a man of my word, as people began to ask questions. Have I lost weight? I deliberately told everyone, yes! To make it sound more specific and challenging, I added my end goal: I'm getting a six-pack! This single sentence that I added at the end made me accountable in front of those people. I wouldn't be able to face them if I didn't deliver on my promise. Now, I have two strong reasons to keep pushing towards my goal. But it didn't stop there. Over time, I developed more reasons that created an even stronger drive. Did you know that less than ten percent of the population has a visible six-pack? On top of my other reasons, I wanted to be part of that ten percent. I'm quite sure this motivation was to boost my self-confidence. The idea was to be different and have something, or be someone special, with something that more than ninety percent of the population don't have and aren't willing to achieve; that's what created this magic pill. Can you see a pattern of addiction? I wanted more and more pills to fuel my drive for success. It's funny how your mind shifts from one thought to another, and that's exactly how this 'pill' was created, starting from a conversation with my lovely wife. We were chatting about one thing, but my mind led me to a compelling reason. The conversation began with how we had already improved our lifestyle and our bodies' new look. My wife mentioned how great it would be to reach forty with our bodies still looking fantastic. I took a moment to analyse the people around me. Only a small fraction of them work on their perfect body or fitness. Gradually, my mind moved to the next reason. Out of everyone I know, I would be one of the few who stood out with a great physique. As a confidence booster, that reason was perfect to add to my list of 'magic pills'. It might sound silly again, but it's about all those reasons that help drive you to reach your goals. Don't be scared or ashamed to be a little selfish, to aim for more, or to want to be better than someone else.

I often wonder, when I see a highly successful person, what their magic pill was. How strong must that secret have been to achieve such vast success, or how many magic pills were needed for that level of achievement? It would be fascinating to understand the true reasons behind what they were willing to sacrifice to realise their dreams. In most cases, the justifications of successful individuals, for you or for me, wouldn't serve as a good example for reaching our own goals. Their minds crafted those reasons, which only hold meaning for them. Looking closely at my surroundings, my wife is an extraordinary example of achieving remarkable goals. She has a very strong magic pill, or at least a hundred magic pills, to achieve what she has achieved so far. She's an ultrarunner. She has completed half-marathons, marathons, and now she faces a real challenge: ultramarathons. For those unfamiliar, an ultramarathon is anything longer than a marathon. I wonder what could be the reason to risk everything to run and finish 150 miles. Yes, that's her latest long-distance race, and she doesn't seem to be stopping there! As I mentioned before, it's incredible what the human body can do when you have a strong purpose, and you are in control of your mind.

Let's return to the idea of having one or more powerful magic pills. For these pills to work like magic and not feel like an extra burden in your routine, but instead naturally drive you to achieve your goals, your body must accept them. To ensure your body accepts these magic pills, your belief plays a crucial role. It's like a form of brainwashing. You need to believe that you genuinely need this. Only by believing in your reasons will your mind adapt and accept what is best for you. Belief creates a natural environment for things to happen on their own. Your mind is amazing and incredibly powerful; it's the best tool you have to learn to harness.

I'll give a perfect example of how most people unconsciously use their minds as tools. My dad, an amazing, hardworking, and very smart person, many years ago would never approve of 4x4 cars in the city. He said, "They are not practical, and they are stupid cars to have!" He had a strong opinion about it, and nothing could change his mind. But now, somehow, it's the best car to have, so what's changed?

Years ago, as a single father and a husband who lost his wife and was the only one in the family responsible for caring for two children, he didn't have time to think about luxury things. The family budget was focused on family priorities. Money was enough to live on, and he always made sure my sister and I had everything, so we never felt like we were missing something. Therefore, things like luxury cars automatically fell to the bottom of the priorities list. It's a simple mental game; I'm pretty sure my dad decided to believe that if something couldn't be afforded, then it wasn't necessary, or even silly. I have my own theory about this, I think it's easier to live that way. There's no pressure to have what you can't afford or don't want. I've seen many times in my life, even myself, doing this, brainwashing ourselves, if you can't afford it, it's not good, or it's stupid. Now, as circumstances have changed and my dad can afford to spend on himself, a 4x4 is the best car to have. It's practical, offers plenty of space, and can get you anywhere.

This is an example of how most people block and unblock their minds based on their needs. With this example, I want you to reflect on what you have previously blocked and now see as essential in your life, or what you are still blocking for good or bad reasons. Unblocking your mind means changing your beliefs to focus on what truly matters for your goals, which helps you think and act without pressure in the right direction.

I had the chance to speak with a few people, all of whom shared the same mindset. They tended to block ideas and come up with reasons why certain things are not good. In these conversations, the main topic was having a visible six-pack, as that was my goal at the time. People's initial response was to explain why they don't need a six-pack, saying it's silly to torture yourself and that it's completely unnecessary. These comments all boil down to "if I don't have it or can't have it, it's bad." If I shared the same mindset, "it's stupid to have a six-pack because I don't have it, or I can't get it", I would never achieve my goal. It's time for you to unblock all those silly, unnecessary blocks and move towards your perfect body mindset.

One of the best exercises for positive thinking and building stronger beliefs is to practise reverse thinking. Focus not on what you can't do or what you don't have, but on what you can do and what you possess. This exercise provides a solid foundation for problem-solving, especially when you know you have a problem and need a solution. Instead of dwelling on what you can't do to resolve your issue, concentrate on what you can do. Likewise, if the problem isn't solvable with what you don't have, focus on what you do have or what you can acquire. It all comes down to having the right mindset. Successful people believe they can attain everything and do anything, so you should think the same to become one of the successful ones.

I used this reversed method on myself. I made up my mind believe that I love something simple like salad. Just plain green leaves, which are often tasteless but great for your diet. I need to keep my calories low, but at the same time, I want to feel full. I've never been a huge fan of salads, but I have found significant benefits from eating them. Large salad portions are low in calories and always surprisingly fill me up.

So, the question is, how do you convince yourself and adapt to the idea that a salad will be an excellent choice? The first benefit is that it's the easiest food to prepare for lunch. Just grab a pack of salads, wash them if needed, and pour them into the bowl. Add some meat or another type of protein, and top it up with your favourite spices. For a tasteless salad, I always use a bit of salt, black pepper, chilli, or smoked pepper. Simple things make a huge difference.

Another good reason to eat salad is that you don't need to think about what you'll have for lunch. Make it a standard low-calorie base for lunch, then add protein and spices to create one complete meal of the day. Eating salads for lunch makes it easier to balance your other meals throughout the day. I'm sure you also agree that quick and lazy meals are more sustainable for you. As soon as you start spending more time deciding what to eat, you'll likely choose something outside of controlled calories, such as a chocolate snack with a decent amount of calories or, even worse, some uncontrolled fast food, simply because it's quick and requires no thought. So, help yourself by making a standard lunch to stay in control.

The third reason to love salads is that they help keep your calorie intake low. I found it difficult initially to know which foods to eat while remaining in a calorie deficit, yet salads are always a premium choice. So, now you have three simple reasons to love salads, but that doesn't mean you need to develop an obsession with them. What I mean is that applying a similar mindset to your thoughts can help you to appreciate things. Give yourself good reasons to start loving things that can positively influence and lead you towards success.

It's a mind game; you trick your mind into wanting what you need, not what you think you like to have. As a small bonus, because you have been good during the main lunch, you can treat yourself to some snacks. Controlled snacks will be your relief and reward. Most importantly, don't restrict yourself by cutting certain foods out of your meals. In a moment when your mind catches you blocking your food desires, you can consider that you lost the battle. So, a solution is to eat everything you desire, but in smaller portions, and whenever possible, replace high-calorie foods with equally low-calorie options, like oven-roasted veggies instead of potato fries. I know it's not the same, but do this from time to time, so you don't get bored with eating veggies all the time. Maintaining this balance is super important because different foods offer different nutrients that your body needs. Even sweets are part of a balanced diet; they mainly help your mind stay calm and settle cravings. For your success and mental relaxation, treat yourself to some controlled guilty pleasure snacks. I believe we should eat everything and avoid restricting entire food categories. Remember to eat everything, but eat less, to stay in a calorie deficit. Your mind will be much calmer as you make these dietary changes.

What are the consequences of not having a magic pill? What is the main reason for achieving your perfect body? I have met many people with different diets and success stories, but once those stories ended, they often reverted to their original habits or became even worse. In these cases, people become confused and less motivated. The problem has always been not having a strong enough reason to drive and sustain success. It should be a rule: don't even think about starting a journey to a perfect body without a solid reason to do it! It sounds harsh, but without a solid reason, you will fail. As you know, failure will only demotivate you and set you back. So, avoid this by having "the very best reason" and start your journey towards success.

Ask yourself: What sparked your idea of a perfect body? Why and how did it happen? Dive deep into these questions. Find your reason, even if it seems silly, stupid, or embarrassing, because these reasons will motivate you on your journey. It's essential to understand the real reason behind your new goal. For example, think of a common situation where someone, a friend, family member, or colleague, accidentally comments or makes a joke about your appearance. You know how people often say things without considering the impact. Try to remember or imagine how you'd feel. Most people might laugh it off or pretend nothing happened, but inside, that comment or joke can linger, causing upset. This is a typical example of how such comments can foster insecurities, leading people to see this as their main issue. I'm sure you can recall similar experiences from your own life. These insecurities often stem from past comments or jokes. I remember a few such moments myself; they linger in my mind and make it hard not to dwell on them. My mind kicks into protection mode, driving me to never encounter that situation or hear that joke again. I realised that this mental 'click' is a self-protection mechanism; the mind switches into survival mode when it perceives danger, whether physical, like injury, or mental, like damage to confidence. In both cases, the mind automatically activates this self-defence. It can either help you or make life more challenging. But how does self-protection work? Both physical and mental threats trigger actions from your mind, which governs your entire body. You'd be surprised at what your mind can do in dangerous situations. Scientific studies show that in life-or-death scenarios, people can push beyond their limits to stay alive. We are endowed with this survival instinct, an incredible asset. However, there's a downside if you're unaware of it: this self-protection can complicate your life. For instance, if you're trying to lose weight drastically, you'll eventually feel hungry. Your brain perceives this as starvation, which triggers the self-protection mode because your body senses danger. It begins storing reserves to ensure your survival. Suddenly, weight loss halts, despite being on a diet, and you might feel confused as to why. One crucial rule is to avoid feeling hungry. Don't give your mind a reason to oppose you. To control your mind, you need to trick it. In this case, having something small to eat, even if it slightly exceeds your daily calorie goal, is wise. The best choice is a large glass of water, as hunger is sometimes just a thirst signal. Drinking water can help satiate you without adding extra calories. Once the hunger signal is blocked, your mind deactivates the self-protection mode, allowing you to resume your weight loss journey. It's incredible how the mind and body collaborate to ensure survival.

I'll provide you with tools to achieve your perfect body, but only you can decide whether to use them. Ask yourself: Is it truly for you? Can you incorporate it into your lifestyle? I'll explain what to expect and what you need to be prepared for throughout your journey. I'll outline how challenging or easy it can be, and how long it might take, but as long as you have your strongest reason, your 'magic pill', you will overcome any obstacle along the way. Unfortunately, magic pills don't look as you might imagine. This magic pill exists, but it resides within you as the best reason to drive you towards success. As an ambitious person, unconsciously, these reasons will motivate you and become part of your daily life. The moment you feel you've achieved your goal, you should have your next strong reason to keep going. I can assure you that you'll find another reason because you'll have tasted the sweetness of success. You'll experience that indescribable feeling of being able to do more and achieve more. Become addicted to your magic pills and enjoy a successful future.

With a new you and magic pills in your pocket, there's no turning back to old habits. That's history. Forget it! It's time to concentrate on your new, brighter future. Focus on where you want to be, not what's easy. This will be a new, better, prouder, healthier, more confident, and more ambitious lifestyle.

Magic pill double-strength supplement

Almost everyone, as children, received life lessons from their parents, especially about using medicine. Most parents never tire of telling you the same thing: if you take medicine, never mix two or more different pills. This sentence has stuck in my mind, and probably yours, since childhood. Of course, it is good advice, except in this particular situation. Forget for a moment what your parents said about mixing pills. This special occasion calls for you to combine these magic pills as much as possible to achieve your dreams. Let's go back to when you were unwell and talking with your parents. After they gave you the pills, what was their next comment? "Make sure you eat plenty of fruit." These parents, with their life lessons, bless them! We all know that fruits are full of vitamins and are always recommended when you're unwell, to boost your immune system and promote a quick recovery. On this point, I completely agree. Your magic pill, the best reason is the one worth dying for, will work very well, but for double the strength, people need an extra boost. For a greater magic effect, every magic pill should be complemented with an additional supplement. This supplement is made from many ingredients, mainly vitamins. It's a double-strength booster designed to help you reach your goals every day. You know, and I know, that vitamins are essential for maintaining health and strength. Most importantly, they are necessary for boosting our immune system. So, to stay healthy and in good shape, you need a small, correct amount of the alphabet of vitamins daily. We are all familiar with vitamins A, B, C, D, and the other nine essential vitamins in the human body. These vitamins play a crucial role in our health. For the best results, combine your magic pills and mix them, but for an extra boost, include your supplement with all its good ingredients. It will be an incredible recipe for better performance and amazing results on your journey to a perfect body.

As you know now, the magic pill is your best reason that's worth dying for, but what is this supplement and all the good ingredients in it? In this case, your daily supplement for double strength will be your discipline. To keep moving forward, discipline is the most important support. Discipline is the best success booster. If you want to be successful in your journey, you must build skills and adapt your discipline level to where your success just happens naturally. As you know, to achieve your perfect body goal, you must be successful, and to be successful, you must be disciplined.

Every point always relates back to your mind. All power and secrets are in control. Control your mind and your thoughts. When you learn to own and govern your mind, everything else becomes amazingly easy. Now you know your supplement, but what about the ingredients? Let's look a bit deeper into these vitamins that create double-strength supplements. What makes discipline durable? The small, good habits in your life, like planning the next steps, routine and consistency, avoiding distraction, self-control, positivity, being healthy, and managing stress. These are your vitamins, and having them in good portions will help you to be disciplined. So, you might ask me, how can I be disciplined? I'll explore these vitamins, the foundation of strong discipline, and explain each vitamin a bit more. I'll give you the first vitamin: how to plan out your goals and the steps to follow. I'll provide examples for you to imagine yourself doing them. You will find some of these steps very familiar, but it's great to have the opportunity to refresh what each means.

First, set a clear goal. Your goal must be specific, measurable, achievable, relevant, and within a defined timeframe. These types of goals, which are proven to be remarkably successful, are called SMART goals. It's usually hard to remember the meaning of each letter in SMART. So, get a pen and a piece of paper, then write down, as simply and briefly as possible, the meaning and actions for each letter, like bullet points. Once you have everything written, make sure this paper is placed somewhere visible, such as on the wall beside your work desk, so that whenever you look up, you see your SMART goal. Another good place is your bedside table, where you can see it every morning or at least once daily as a reminder of your goal. On a humorous note, stick this paper with your clear bullet points in your bathroom. The best spot is a wall or door facing the toilet. When you're resting or on duty, trust me, you won't miss it.

So, returning to the meaning of each letter, the first letter S will stand for specific. You must be truly clear about your goal description. It should be detailed enough to avoid misunderstandings or leading yourself into a grey area. For these reasons, you must eliminate options to escape when things get tough. So, your goal will be for you to achieve your perfect body. It obviously won't be a vague description. The common idea of a perfect body is a lean and muscular physique. Therefore, the first step and goal would be to lose weight. Remember to be specific, such as saying: "I want to lose weight, but I only want to reduce my body fat percentage, and I don't want to lose muscle mass." This clearly states what you want to happen in your weight loss goal. With this sentence, you are clear and specific about how you want the final result to look.

The second letter M will stand for measurable. You will need a clear, measurable end point. This will normally be a number for what you will be setting up for you to achieve. The moment you see this number will be the moment you achieve your goal. For example, to look lean, a man set a goal to achieve a body fat percentage of 15%, but for women its hilly higher, 20%. Of Corse these numbers are average, for every person it will be slightly different. These are noticeably clear numbers to aim for. For some people, these numbers probably mean nothing. So, I suggest you do some research on how the body approximately looks based on these numbers and choose the numbers that best fit you.

The third letter A will stand for achievable. Your goal must be genuinely achievable because something impossible will lead you to failure. Ask yourself whether you have everything needed to achieve your goal. You need tools like mindset, knowledge, and motivation to realistically attain your goal. The answer should be yes; now you have all that you need. Your next point could be something like: My goal is achievable because I have my magic pills, I know what to do and what I need to reach my goal. For motivation, use something like "not a nice problem to have". I don't want to be overweight, struggle to move, be unhappy, or in the worst case, be sick and die. If other people can do that, then why can't I? I'm not worse than them!

The fourth letter R stands for relevant. It should be something you need, and that helps you to change your life. Returning to the questions: Is a perfect body relevant to me? Do I want to look and feel good? Do I want to be healthier? Do I want a magic pill to do the magic for me? There are many questions to answer, but all these things are life-changing and relevant to your goal of achieving a perfect body. So, is it relevant to you? Yes! You are reading this book, and that effort indicates it's very relevant for you.

The last fifth letter, T, will stand for time-bound. Time will be a year, a month, or some special day. There must be a due date for completion so you can pace your efforts. You will set up an endpoint for your target achievement. For example, you want to achieve a perfect body look for your beach holiday. It's been booked for next year in August, or you want to look fabulous at your wedding that has been planned for eighteen months, on the 28th of March. In these examples, I gave you longer timeframes than most people would want. Normally, people want to see final results quickly, in about one to three months, and have the job done. Unfortunately, in most cases, it doesn't work like that. The body needs time to adjust to any new changes, so set up a time frame where you gradually and consistently lose weight. Give as reasonable a time frame as possible to avoid failure and to succeed in your journey. To achieve your perfect body look, you will need to give yourself more time; don't rush, take the time for greater results. Time is necessary for your body to adapt and adjust. Changes must be as healthy as possible, and you must be careful to avoid creating other health issues. Rushing through quick weight loss can easily harm you. For example, not consuming enough vitamins to maintain a good immune system or not having enough calories throughout the day could make you feel powerless and weak. What are the consequences of a low immune system? In the best case, you could injure yourself, perhaps minor injuries like tripping, falling, losing focus, or bruising, or even a dislocated body part. What if you are not so lucky? In the worst case, it could be 'Game Over': you might become very sick, and your health could be seriously damaged. It could even cause you to forget about the dream of your perfect body for a long time. Love yourself and look after yourself; give your body time to adjust to changes slowly.

This vitamin, "planning out your SMART goals", will help you maintain your discipline easily with clear and straightforward steps. One of the main rules of discipline is that actions should be clear so you know what to do and where to focus, avoiding wasted time on rethinking, reinventing, and failing. A lack of discipline stems from a lack of clarity; making each goal as clear as possible and sticking to it is essential.

Do you know what works very well? Things that happen automatically, like what would be programmed in your mind. Daily tasks you do, and later in the day, you try to remember whether they're done. These tasks happen without conscious thought throughout the day. What can help improve discipline? Habits and routines are your foundation! The next vitamins that MUST be in your supplement recipe are good habits and routines. There are much better chances for you to achieve your goals if you don't need to think about it; it's just done. Having good habits combined with a routine can do miracles, like counting calories and doing that every single time before you put food in your mouth, doing activities, and sticking to set days and times to avoid second thoughts or the habit of eating healthily. When you shop, only visit aisles and shelves packed with healthy products. Make a shopping route to follow; whenever you are in the shop, you will avoid aisles with things that you really don't need. The best thing about this habit and routine is that it eliminates the temptation for unhealthy stuff. I started my route through the aisles when my wife and I decided to avoid occasional alcohol use. Most of us know that feeling of being tempted to grab a beer or wine for dinner or to watch a movie. The simple idea is that if you don't have it, you can't use it. With this habit and routine, I fixed the root cause of my problem of occasionally having an alcoholic drink.

The routine will give you that feeling that is so needed in the perfect body journey; it will be your freedom. You will have set days and times for all daily tasks, and without thinking, you will just do them. The hardest part is creating a plan and starting it, but now, with all the routine plans in place and set up, it becomes as easy as possible. Routines are based on consistency. Just stick to the schedule as closely as you can. A routine is a great tool for someone struggling mentally with daily tasks. With routine help, you can establish eating times, for example, you like to eat three times a day. Your breakfast will be every weekday morning at seven o'clock. Lunch is set at twelve o'clock, and dinner at five o'clock. These times allow roughly five hours between meals. A five-hour gap is reasonable for food consumption. Prepare yourself; it will feel like forever at first, but that's only because we're so used to snacking whenever we want. We don't need to keep ourselves busy with eating; we eat because we have free time and food nearby. Another reason for constant snacking is boredom, and we entertain ourselves with tasty snacks. It sounds ridiculous, but it's true. On days when you are busy with things like last-minute tasks before the family arrives or when you've completely lost track of time with your hobby, you will find yourself eating less. Instead of filling dull or unproductive moments with snacks, your mind is too occupied to process urgent or interesting things. To keep yourself away from snacks, find something that interests you and keep your mind busy with hobbies and physical activities. Find something you enjoy, or that makes you happy.

Let's explore the twenty-first century's most essential vitamin. Living in this century, most of us are trapped by numerous distractions. The most common is social media. We all try to benefit from rich and overwhelming information, but we forget how much it distracts us from what we should focus on and the tasks that must be completed. Spending hours online, we steal our most precious resource: time. Therefore, having the next vitamin for stronger discipline will help focus your mindset on clear goals and provide more personal time. Minimising distractions could solve around thirty percent of your problems. Living nowadays is both easy and hard. It's easy because access is everywhere, wherever you look, whatever you're doing, entertainment is at your fingertips. Yet, it's hard because, in the back of our minds, we realise we are trapped without a time limit. Sometimes, you catch yourself spending hours on your phone, flipping through articles, videos, news, or just watching movies, only to realise you've wasted all this time instead of focusing on something productive and useful. I support the idea of maintaining balance in everything you do. Yes, social media can be a distraction, and yes, you should control how much time you spend on it, but nowadays, staying aware of current events and not being like a caveman is necessary. It's beneficial to be mindful of popular topics and to educate yourself on the latest discoveries worldwide and new technologies that can make our lives easier and safer. To boost your confidence, knowing and understanding what's happening around the world makes you an interesting person to converse with. People will want to approach and talk to you because there will always be topics to discuss and share thoughts about. Now, let's consider the consequences, my favourite topic. Recognising consequences broadens your understanding of how badly things can go wrong and illustrates the importance of respecting certain boundaries. Being trapped on social media makes you forget your routine, your plans, and your goals because you're entertained and having fun. This automatically makes you lazy, skipping your physical activities, indulging in snacks, and forgetting your goals. It all begins with a quick snack or break to see what's new in the world, but it never stops there. Soon, you're scrolling through random articles or videos, finding them interesting, and instead of doing your physical activity, you spend more time on social media. And what's the best thing to have when you're entertained? Yes, some naughty snacks. After indulging in these treats, you feel tired, and your goals seem less important. It's so easy to slip down the hill amid today's distractions. Use social media wisely and stay informed about the world, but remember to control yourself.

Mentioning control over ourselves leads me to the next vitamin, "Self-control." Self-control is another valuable tool to help you stay as disciplined as possible. Most often, people act impulsively, and those moments are when they lose control. For a successful fitness journey, self-control is crucial; temptation plays a significant role in everyday life. For example, snacking is the biggest obstacle for many in keeping their daily calories in deficit, but if you learn to say NO and resist temptation, your problem is half solved, bringing you one step closer to your ideal body. Each time you feel like opening the fridge or cupboard and reaching for a snack, STOP and THINK. Do you really need that snack, or is it just in your mind? I bet that in ninety-five percent of cases, when you reach for a snack, you actually don't need it, at least not with a good reason. It's just a habit because you can, and because you have a choice. The best way to combat temptation is to remove the choice. As I already mentioned, if you don't keep snacks in your cupboard or fridge, but only food for preparing your next meals, you eliminate the possibility of grabbing a quick snack. When shopping, skip the snack aisles; if you don't have snacks around, you won't eat them, simple as that!

The other five percent of why you reach for a snack could be due to a reasonable reason, like experiencing weakness or cravings, which might mean your body needs a quick sugar boost for energy. In such cases, the best approach is to listen to your body and choose that snack. However, be cautious with this, as it can quickly become an excuse to snack frequently. Do not use it as a justification for cheating, because you are only deceiving yourself and harming only yourself.

Home and places where the environment is under your control can be easier to manage, but what about situations where control is not in your hands? For example, when snacks are around you, and you can't avoid the choice of having them, like in your workplace, which is outside your control zone. It's a day when your colleague has his birthday. As a kind gesture, your colleague brings plenty of tasty-looking snacks and places them on the table next to the door exit, and you must pass this table every single time you leave the room. You have this irritating feeling; each time you pass this table, these delicious-looking snacks seem to speak to you. These snacks tempt you, showing how good and tasty they are, but you are on your perfect body journey, and the temptation to reach for one is enormous each time you pass by. Having those snacks might seem to calm your mind, which remains alert about these sweets. It's all in your mind, and you must learn how to take charge of your thoughts.

When temptation is strong, it is easy to act impulsively and let your mind switch off, leading you straight to consequences. There's always this thought in the back of your mind: I'll be a little naughty just this once, and I'll act better tomorrow. But will you? With self-control, you can stop being weak and vulnerable. Remember, in those moments when you feel you're starting to lose control, you have your magic pill, you have "your best reason that's worth dying for" which can give you the power to say no. Catch that moment before you act impulsively: just stop yourself and think about what is more important. Practising this will make it easier over time. The easier it gets, the stronger you become mentally. You will start to feel in control and make decisions because you'll gradually gain confidence. Mainly, self-control is needed for two things: first, controlling what you eat; second, pushing yourself to engage in physical activities. Once you master these two, everything else in life will begin to fall into place, just as you wish. Unconsciously, you will be in control of your decisions and actions.

Like everything else in our lives, discipline needs positivity. Imagine vitamins that boost your positive mindset. You can only gain this discipline power through positive thoughts. The first step to having positive thoughts and maintaining positivity is to look around and observe the kind of people you are surrounded by. As humans, we are very easily influenced by those around us. For example, if you have work colleagues who are unhappy with their jobs and constantly complain about how bad the workplace is, you will automatically start to feel the same negative emotions, even if you previously loved your job and workplace. I have personally learned not to focus on such people because their negativity can drain you. Sadly, there will always be someone negative around you, and they can become barriers to your success. Phrases like, "NO, " "I CAN'T, " "DO YOU REALLY NEED THAT," "WHY ARE YOU TORTURING YOURSELF," "DON'T YOU HAVE BETTER THINGS TO DO," or "THAT'S STUPID," are common expressions of negativity. These phrases reflect negativity, judgement, lack of belief, and no support. You will become more mentally disciplined if you avoid hearing such comments. So, help yourself: ignore and steer clear of all that negativity.

Let's imagine the opposite scenario. This time, you are the person at work who is unhappy with the new job duties, but all colleagues are fantastic people with positive minds, and it's nice to see and be around them every day. How would that make you feel? In the beginning, you might have mixed feelings about your job because you dislike the work itself but enjoy the environment. This makes it very difficult to leave the place. Positivity attracts people, but negativity traps them. Think about those living on a positive wave, who are happy to see you and inspire you to improve your life. Stick with people who truly wish you all the best and support you with new and challenging ideas for a better future. In conversations with people in your circle, you can tell who genuinely wants you to be happy and successful. From those people, you will receive support, encouragement, and belief in you, no judgment, no matter how crazy your ideas may be. Often, you'll find similar ideas and life goals with these people, so stay with them and help each other become better versions of yourselves.

Remember, this works both ways, just like in every relationship. You can't expect everyone to be positive and supportive all the time, but you might be sceptical and forget to give support and a positive attitude in return. To keep people around who support and inspire you, rather than bring you down, you must do the same; you need to put effort into them. Encourage them with your achievements, stories, and reasons for a better life because ambitious and successful people with dreams and goals won't tolerate negativity around them; they are smart enough to know that only positive thoughts lead to success. For extra help in achieving your perfect body journey, find people who share your positive mindset and body goals, and perhaps even have healthy competition to boost your motivation. Keep them close, there's always something to talk about, whether it's sharing experiences or exchanging useful tips. Get inspired by others' positive success stories and share your own to build stronger relationships with disciplined-minded individuals, because success stories are built on consistent positive discipline.

To maintain good and consistent discipline, you must have one more crucial thing to look after: your health. People sometimes forget to take care of themselves, which can quickly lead to disaster. You must remember to preserve your health and well-being. It's important on your journey to a perfect body because your body will change. As your body improves and transforms, you will notice and feel how it gets better and stronger. However, your body can become a little fragile during this process. Before it gets stronger, it may become somewhat weaker, and these are the moments when you must look after yourself and treat yourself to extra rest or healthy food rich in real vitamins. To uphold good discipline, you must be disciplined in maintaining high standards of health and well-being. Health and discipline go hand in hand like a magic circle. To stay disciplined, you need energy, focus, and drive, but to have those, you need good health so your body can improve. Our bodies are designed to be active, and the more active they are, the healthier and stronger they become. Every health specialist would tell you the same: you need regular exercise, and with regular exercise, you must ensure you get enough sleep and eat as healthy as possible for your body to have the best recovery. If your body has good recovery, you will have good levels of energy, and you will be able to focus towards achieving your goals. Your body will feel stronger and more capable of facing new challenges, leading to that wonderful feeling of well-being, energy, and happiness. To enjoy these benefits, you must stick to discipline. Continue with regular exercise, ensure you sleep well, and eat properly and healthily.

Unfortunately, being healthy isn't enough with just exercise, good sleep, and great food. The biggest threat to our health, as everyone knows, is bad stress. To maintain good well-being, your stress levels must be managed. I'm talking about being in control of how bad stress affects your life. Let's look at the consequences of living with constant stress. First, stress distracts you from your goals because it takes over your thoughts, making it hard to think clearly, and your goals become less important. Second, bad stress can lead to serious health issues. It kind of harms you from within; your body focuses only on stress and forgets to protect itself. Most people find that stress is a root cause of their health problems. The benefits of managing stress will be incredible, and you'll start to notice them very quickly once you sort out bad stress from your life. Stress has this remarkably negative strength. It can distract you, no matter where you are, what you do, or how you feel. If you live a stressful lifestyle, stress will dominate every single thought or feeling. Without this stress-free 'vitamin,' your double-strength supplement will never work as a magic pill because stress will take over and become the main, if not the only, thought in your mind. No matter how good all the other vitamins are, in just a split second, stress can easily distract you from planning your goals, causing you to stop following your daily routine and forget about self-control and consistency. With stress, there is no room for positivity because your mind will focus on what worries you. However, you might be tempted to find relief in social media nonsense, which only makes you feel calmer for a moment. Stress will overpower your strict discipline if you don't manage it. For discipline to work and be effective, you need a clear mind. As with all your problems, stress resides in your mind. When you learn to control your mind, you can control your stress and allow your mind to focus on positive things.

How you look and feel being addicted.

Being addicted to something often seems like a negative thing. When you hear about a person being addicted, the first thing in your mind will be, "bad habit addiction", like alcohol, drug, or gambling addictions. However, addiction is not always harmful; it depends on what kind of addiction we discuss. In this case, addiction to these magic pills isn't negative at all. Ask yourself: how can being addicted to success be bad? Of course, moderation is key because too much of anything isn't good. But your commitment to having strong reasons for your goals will help turn your dreams into reality. If you can use this addiction to achieve your ideal body, just imagine how impressive that would be. To ensure you reach this impressive look, I'll give you one extra tip: find pictures of different perfect-looking body types. Choose the image that best represents your dream physique and set it as your visual goal. Everyone needs a clear idea of what their end goal should look like. This will give you an additional way to compare and ask yourself: "Am I there yet?" Among all options, select the one that suits you best. Don't be afraid to decide how you want to look. It could be shredded, athletic, bulky, or even slim. Everyone's idea of a perfect body is different, but focus on what your dream body would look like.

You have a clear visual goal, but now let's talk about the feelings that come with your perfect body. Have you ever considered how people feel about achieving those perfect bodies? One reason is to look great. With your perfect body, you will get extra benefits. Your confidence boost will be through the roof, but it's not finished there. Your body will feel tight and strong, not flimsy and weak. That's the recipe for an unstoppable and successful person. It's amazing when the body begins to transform. The first time I felt my midsection be incredibly tight and strong, it made me realise how wonderful that feeling is. It was the complete opposite of how I felt before starting the perfect body journey. We all know and dislike that feeling when your belly, chest, and love handles jiggle up and down during brisk walking. That has always been a red flag for me, but it was never a good enough reason to do something about it. When you start seeing and feeling improvements in your body, it gives you that extra motivation to go further. Naturally, you'll want to keep pushing for better results.

My goal has always been to achieve a visible six-pack. I have a clear picture of how I want my six-pack to look. While researching ways to develop a perfectly sculpted six-pack, I learned that not everyone can have all six bottom blocks visible. Due to different physiques, some people can only have their upper abs visible. Many bodybuilders, despite their efforts, could never achieve a perfectly visible six-pack with all six blocks. That was a shock to me! I always imagined myself with a perfect six-pack. It is hard to accept that I may never attain the look I visualised.

Throughout my journey to achieve a lean physique, I finally reached that final stage where only a small stubborn patch of belly fat remained, and all my worries faded. One day, after a gym session, I unintentionally startled and confused my wife. It wasn't deliberate, but my message came out wrong. I told her: "Today, I felt something on my body!" Her first thought was, it doesn't sound good, it's something bad. At the same time, I didn't seem worried; on the contrary, I was overly excited, which confused her further. I saw her confusion and panic in her eyes, so I hurried to explain. After working hard on my abs during the session, my midsection was very pumped and felt strong. When I was about to shower, I checked myself in the mirror, as everyone does, mainly to confirm my progress. I pressed my hand to the lower abdomen, just below the last bit of stubborn belly fat I was trying to lose, and felt those two abs blocks at last. The hardest to develop are the lower abdomen blocks, which I had wondered if

I would ever see in my six-pack. That silly excitement motivated me to push even harder. It felt like I could see the light at the end of the tunnel. The lesson here is that things don't always go as planned. While you can imagine a certain look, genetics may prevent it from happening. The key is not to give up but to learn to appreciate what you have and adapt your goals accordingly. If luck is on your side and everything aligns, celebrate it as a boost to motivate yourself even more. Looking in the mirror and liking what you see is a fantastic feeling.

What describes healthy and ambitious people? Good energy, consistency, willpower, and a strong drive. That's how you will look and feel being addicted. You will often find yourself with low energy, feeling like you "can't be bothered". Without energy, your success will diminish, but there are always options, and you always have the choice to be full of energy because, like everything else, it is in your mind. It's great to be full of positive energy, able to go and do things, and feel unstoppable. With consistency and a will to act, people around you will see you as a doer. With a doer image, you will start to appear more successful, and from that feeling, you will become successful. A strong drive will help you finish what you started and create a fulfilling sense of accomplishment.

Find what you love. Everyone has a part of their body that they adore. While scrolling through pictures of perfect body types, I fell in love with a specific area. In fact, the most difficult body part to make lean and muscular enough to be visible is the lower abdominal muscles, commonly known as the lower abs. I consider it "the sexiest part of the body." This flat, tight area on your body reveals a lot about you. From personal experience, reaching that point is extremely challenging, and maintaining it is even harder. Everyone has a particular body part or area on a well-trained, lean body that they find most attractive. It could be for one person shoulder and back, and for another person chest, arms, or for someone just legs. Someone might find the entire upper body quite appealing, especially men with that V-shape, which looks very masculine. The middle section, the six-pack, is incredibly attractive for anyone to have. Enthusiasts of the lower body might get excited about muscular legs or glutes; for example, calf muscles can be a focus because, especially in summer when wearing shorts, they are visible and can look very sexy. I challenge you to choose the most attractive part or area of your body and imagine it perfectly shaped. So, fall in love with your body, feel fantastic, and develop a fondness for yourself.

So, a picture with a clear end goal will help you better see where you stand at the end of your ideal body journey. Use this picture to compare and see how far or close you are to your goal. Don't be afraid to fall in love with this one particular part or area of your body, since you will be motivated to make this area as perfect as possible, and in doing so, everything else will improve. You want to become addicted to these magic pills, these incredibly strong reasons that will lead you to any success.

Have you been diagnosed correctly?

What happens when the diagnosis of your problem is wrong? Simply put, it can lead to failure or cause other issues. For pills to work, we must identify the real problem to achieve a successful outcome. It's important to understand what you want as your end goal. Know which direction to take to avoid misunderstanding and to be successful. It is easy to fail if you go in the wrong direction from your goal or if you believe you are doing the right things for the wrong reasons. Often, I come across people who have no idea or only basic information about how to start a perfect body journey. There is one fundamental thing that people often mix up. You can eat healthily and live healthily, but that doesn't guarantee you will reach your perfect body.

In my eyes, there are three types of diagnoses in a perfect body journey. On this point, try to understand the correct diagnosis for your problem.

The first type of diagnosis will be for people who like the idea of a healthier lifestyle and weight loss, but it stops there. For them, it's always just a great idea and nothing more. The first type of people don't want to put in any effort, and they don't want that hassle. Most of the time, these people are not ambitious; they like things the way they are. For people to be honest with themselves and realise what they're capable of and what their priorities are in their busy lives is one of the first starting points. These people will be okay with what they look like because, for them, how they look will be at the bottom of the priority list. Don't torture yourself with goals that are not important for you or what's not important for that moment. For this diagnosis, people must learn to love themselves as they are. With wrong goals at the wrong time, you will lead yourself to failure, and failure will lead to low morale and disappointment.

Two other types of diagnosed individuals always desire more from life. You are reading this book to research how to achieve your perfect body, so you are certainly not the first type of person. It's a good idea to be healthy and shed some weight, but the first type of person can't be bothered, because they are happy with themselves as they are. You want more from life, and you're ready to do more. You have ambition, but now you need to clarify which of the two other types of diagnoses you fall into.

So, ask a question!

Do you want to be a healthy person and live a healthy lifestyle? If the answer is yes, go for it! Every scientific study proves that healthy lifestyles lead to better and longer lives. Just live your life as healthily as possible and enjoy it. Eat healthily and stay active; that's all you need. Off thinking, "I'm doing everything that counts as healthy," can make you feel good. That feeling could be enough for your mind to be happy. If your mind is happy and calm, you will be pleased with your appearance and your life. This lifestyle requires a small amount of ambition, which most people have. Type two diagnosed people will be ready to do a bit more than nothing to live a happy and healthy lifestyle. It's a small effort for satisfactory results.

Type three diagnosed individuals want to be healthy, but also seek a perfect body look. These individuals are highly ambitious. Their ambition always remains a top priority. They aim to succeed in any way possible, often achieving success because they have the best reason that's worth dying for, and because of this, they will do whatever it takes to reach all their goals. They possess many powerful 'magic pills' in their back pocket and have a strong addiction to them.

These individuals are always prepared to do more and think differently because they possess the magic pill that drives them. Many people fall into this third category because they care a little more about themselves and how others perceive them. I must admit, I am one of them. I want to be healthy, but I also want to accomplish something that most people can't. "Can't" is not quite right; let me correct myself: they "don't want to", because it's difficult. People dislike difficulty. We live in a time where everything is made simpler, and we are so accustomed to this lifestyle. It's easy to do nothing, sit on the sofa, watch TV, eat, and become overweight. But you are not that person! You have a powerful tool, your mind, and you will change your life so that you can look and feel motivated by success.

Make sure to understand which diagnosis you have to avoid unnecessary failures. If you're still unsure, I'll tell you. You are diagnosed with the ambition to be successful! You want to be healthy with a perfect body, full of energy and driven to achieve your goals.

How to swallow a pill

The magic pill won't work without instructions. Everyone would agree that leaving this pill on the bedside table and hoping it will start working is a complete failure. As we all know, for the pill to work, you must swallow it. For the magic pill to be effective, you need to take some action. For medicine to heal, you must enter it into your body or have it applied to your body, and for that, as we know, some action is required. In this case, you have your magical pill, and you will need to swallow it. For some people, this can be a problem because not everyone can swallow pills without difficulty. It is not a simple action for everyone, and the reasons can include fear of swallowing because it might get stuck in the throat, not knowing how to swallow because they have never done it before, or simply not having the right things around them, such as a glass of water.

You had a problem, found a way to speak with your doctor, and now you have a prescription with what seem like magical pills as a solution. You're back home from the pharmacy with a bag full of your medication. Typically, before people take a pill, they ask questions and try to find answers. These answers are usually written in the medicine manual that comes with the packaging. The manual usually starts with some information that most people prefer not to know and rarely read. This time, it will be no different; you can skip this initial part of the manual, but I'll give you a quick shortcut. So, I'll provide all that long and complicated information in a short, clear, and understandable version.

I always begin with these magic pills that will help with your problems. In your case, your issue is reaching your ideal body; whether it involves losing or gaining some weight, you'll need to follow certain rules. The main rule is to establish an 80/20 routine. Eighty percent of it will be your diet, and twenty percent will be physical activity. This depends on your goal, but since most people want to lose weight, let's say eighty percent of your focus should be on maintaining a calorie deficit. Simply put, you consume fewer calories than you burn. To achieve this, unfortunately, you need to count every single calorie you consume, including every piece of food or liquid you put in your mouth. You probably have heard the saying "Abs are made in the kitchen". Before I seriously embarked on the journey to my perfect body, I didn't understand this saying. However, after some time, I witnessed my own body transformation by following this phrase.

People usually discuss weight loss, but what about those whose aim is to gain weight? Many don't realise that some individuals struggle to add extra mass. So, if you need to increase your weight, follow this same method: track your calories, but ensure you eat more than you burn. Avoid filling up on easy calories from fatty, processed foods. They contribute to fat, not muscle!

1. How many pills should I take, and how often?

2. What should I do with this pill?

3. How long will it take before you start seeing some results?

4. When should I take the first pill?

These are likely the first questions on your mind when you have your pills in hand. It's all about following instructions to stay safe and recover as quickly as possible. The beauty of these magic pills is that you can't overdose on them. So, in answer to the first question, you can take as many as you need and as often as you need to start seeing results. Having these magic pills, as many as you want and as frequently as you can, I don't see any harm or health risks involved. Start with this single pill, your one best reason, for some time; if it works, you probably won't need more pills. But if you find it's not strong enough and you need an extra dose, go ahead and get the next pill straight away and have your next best reason to proceed.

For the second question, about what to do with this pill, the answer is simple: swallow it! (Find your "The best reason". The reason why you will do anything to achieve your goal.) This medication is in pill form, and as we generally know, pills are typically taken orally, so this one should be used the same way. To swallow this magical pill, you will need to prepare first. That means performing a few steps. To do this, get a glass, find the tap with fresh water, and fill the glass. Once prepared, take the magical pill, place it in your mouth, drink a glass of water, and swallow. These are straightforward actions, especially if you follow the guidelines and step-by-step instructions; all you need to do is simply follow them.

Let's do some preparation work before you're ready to swallow the magic pill. Like getting a glass of water, you will need to gather very essential tools for your perfect body journey. I'll provide a step-by-step list of what to do and what kind of tools you will need for your success.

The first step is to get a small kitchen scale, similar to getting a glass. As I mentioned, abs are made in the kitchen, and your entire journey to a perfect body will revolve around the kitchen. If you don't have one, order it online or buy it from the shop. Choose one with the idea that you're treating yourself to an extra kitchen tool to make your life easier. It will increase pressure on your mind if these changes seem challenging to overcome, and if you feel like taking on an extra task. Once you have these excellent new kitchen scales, keep them somewhere handy, where you can easily reach them without thinking. Every time you prepare food, the scales should be next to you. The best place is on your kitchen counter, where you are usually preparing food, within easy reach. Make it possible to grab a scale without moving your body around the kitchen. Very quickly, this habit will become so automatic that you do it without thinking. I think it's brilliant, one less thing to learn and worry about.

You have a glass, and now you need to find a tap from which to get water. The second step will be a challenge for most people. It will be the thought process: now I must weigh every piece of food before cooking or eating. The first thing in your mind might be: 'It's not for me,' 'I don't have time for that,' or 'I can't be bothered to do that!' Believe me, I've been there! I was once like you, and it took me a while to get through it. Honestly, it took a couple of months to accept this idea. My goal was to lose body fat to reveal my abs. I thought that if I just went to the gym, I would achieve my perfect body. I was so wrong! Hard work in the gym without results left me disappointed and confused. My wife gently suggested a few times that if I wanted to lose weight, the only way was to count calories and stay in a calorie deficit. I held onto this stubborn mindset that I'd rather work hard at the gym than count calories, but I was smart enough to understand that if something doesn't work, you need to change your approach. So, I started researching how to get my perfect body. After reading and watching hundreds of articles and videos, I found one common theme, which is what my wife had been telling me: if you want to lose weight, you must be in a calorie deficit. I am someone who values facts and evidence. So, if everyone, from professional trainers and influencers to doctors and athletes, agrees on the same method for losing weight, it's enough for me. The strongest evidence was right before my eyes: my wife. She had been counting calories all along, lost a good portion of weight, and looked very slim and fit. Seeing her impressive results was enough to convince me. I learned from her and started to weigh every piece of food and count calories to stay in a calorie deficit. She inspired me to start counting calories, and it became our shared goal. Make it as simple and enjoyable as possible so it works. It's easier to do together with your partner, turning it into a topic to talk about, like sharing a hobby.

You have your glass and find a tap; the third step is to turn on the tap. The easiest thing to do. So, as simple as it is, you'll need to download an app. To count and know how many calories you've eaten and how many you can still consume, you need a food tracker app, an app on your smartphone made for calorie counting. It's very handy to have your app on your phone because, let's be honest, your phone goes everywhere with you, so it's always close by. These apps are designed for easy setup and straightforward food tracking. Download the app, set up all the required parameters, and it will then calculate your daily total calories, what you can eat, and help you plan each meal. This calorie-tracking app's effectiveness depends on your discipline. If you input incorrect information, you will get inaccurate calculations, leading to misleading results. To start using this app effectively, you need to prove that you can stay disciplined. The only rule for this app to help you is to track every single food and drink you consume! I'll give an example of how easy it is to overlook calories in routine actions that don't seem to affect your body. Consider some daily activities, such as drinking coffee or tea. Many people wouldn't bother to add these drinks to their tracker because plain ground coffee and tea are calorie-free. However, everything changes when you like your coffee or tea with a small splash of milk. That small splash, about 20ml, depending on the milk's fat content, will be around 10-15 calories. If you add a teaspoon of sugar for sweetness, that's approximately 17 calories. Although it seems minimal for a single drink, many people develop a habit of drinking hot beverages multiple times a day. Now, let's estimate the total daily calories for someone who loves hot drinks as a routine. Suppose this person enjoys milky, sweet coffee with two teaspoons of sugar and a splash of milk, preferring not to drink black, bitter coffee. Most of the time, there's also a simple biscuit or two, accompanying the coffee, forming a typical coffee break. Calculating calories from just one coffee break: ground coffee itself is calorie-free; milk adds about 13 calories; two teaspoons of sugar bring in around 34 calories; and three biscuits could add about 120 calories. This sums up to roughly 167 calories per coffee break. If this person has three such breaks daily, that's a total of 501 calories, equivalent to a quarter of their recommended daily intake. How many such hot drinks do you have in a day? These are empty calories that can make you feel as if you've not eaten at all. It's easy to overlook how quickly calories accumulate through a normal day. With this in mind, your goal to maintain an ideal body should motivate you to manage your calorie intake more carefully.

 The next two steps in this process are to get that pill into your body, which will require some physical movement. Put the pill in your mouth, then drink it with a glass of water. As part of your journey towards a better body, physical activity will play an important role, just like when you engage your biceps to lift a glass of water. People's bodies are built to move and burn calories, but these days, everything around us has been made easier, so we don't need to move much. We can be lazy and comfortable as much as we want. However, we must understand that sitting and doing nothing will harm both our physical health and mental well-being. Even a small amount of physical activity at the start will be enough to begin improving your body.

Just to be clear, doing only physical activities will not help you reach your ideal body goal. Yes, people need to be active, and yes, they need to burn calories, but that is only one part of your journey towards the perfect body. I learned this the hard way. I was mistaken in thinking that hard work and sweating in the gym would be enough to shape my ideal body. Let me tell you the harsh truth: I believe and I stand by it that only about twenty percent of your focus should be on physical activities, while the remaining eighty percent should be on your food and drinks. I initially did it the other way round. I devoted 80% of my effort to the gym and only 20% to my diet. And guess what? No progress at all! I couldn't understand why I was working so hard but seeing no results. I was in the gym, sweating and pushing myself to the limit, and yet nothing changed! The issue was that I was consuming more calories than I burned. It's astonishing how easy it is to eat 2-4 thousand calories a day, but how difficult it is to burn at least one thousand calories. You'd need hours of intensive training to burn all those extra calories. Most people don't have the time or motivation to spend hours every day on physical activities, and you don't have to, but what you do need is some physical activity at least two or three times a week.

For me, physical activity is the gym. It's one of the easiest activities you can find. Gyms are now so accessible to everyone. You can find one pretty easily within your price range and close to your home. If you truly want to find your magic pill, you will choose the best fit for you and take every workout very seriously, because your best reason worth dying for will drive you to succeed. The effort you put into your physical activity will remind you of how difficult it is to burn a few calories. A simple and effective reminder for me is a warm-up, such as running on a treadmill before weight training. I need to run for twenty minutes on the treadmill at a fast pace and incline to remind myself how hard I need to work to earn a chocolate bar. That one chocolate bar, containing three hundred calories, feels like twenty minutes of hell on the treadmill.

Resistance training is proven to be one of the best ways to achieve a perfect body, but if you don't enjoy going to the gym, don't do it. Do something you like. If not the gym, at least ensure it's a physically active exercise. You could go for a run, attend a gym class, play some sports, or find an activity you enjoy. An activity you like will increase your chances of sticking with it. Some activities can be challenging, unpleasant, or not enjoyable, but if you like your chosen activity, you will do it with a smile on your face. Physical activity is, and must be, part of the journey to a perfect body.

What do you need for physical activity? The honest answer is not much. First, you need to decide which physical activity suits you and your lifestyle. Second, you'll need sportswear. If you want to get a new outfit, go ahead, you can start this journey with a confidence boost. For motivation, good-fitting and stylish clothes will play a crucial role. Make sure your sports clothes fit well; they shouldn't be too tight or too loose. Choose an outfit in your favourite colour and design, whatever gives you that feeling, the feeling when you are at your most confident. I actually dare you to have that feeling! Share your confidence and excitement about how good you look and feel as someone who has made exercise part of their lifestyle. The same applies to trainers: pick some nice, colourful and comfortable ones, those dream sports trainers. Treat yourself! You deserve it. You're starting a new chapter. It will give you that "new me" feeling.

Having more tracking methods for your body transformation will give you better data to analyse, and from this data, you can determine what you have done correctly or incorrectly. That will allow you to improve and lead you to success. I have created a habit. I bought one of those smart weight scales and weigh myself every morning. Weighing and tracking myself helps me understand if I am progressing, maintaining, or not improving.

I suggest you try weighing yourself each morning and decide if this method suits you. Different people prefer different approaches; some will prefer weighing themselves every morning, while others will weigh themselves once a week. It all depends on how mentally resilient you are to weight fluctuations. Be prepared for your weight to go down and up almost every morning. Even if you strictly follow your calorie deficit plan, your weight will fluctuate in both directions. Many factors influence your weight. One reason could be that you are exceeding your daily calorie allowance. Another might be that you ate too late in the day or had a heavy combination of foods like bread and meat, which will take longer to digest. Remember, if you are too aggressive in losing weight, your body may make things difficult by switching to self-protection functions and beginning to create reserves to survive. This can happen if you don't consume enough calories for your body to burn or if your body perceives a lack of energy.

Try to handle your ups and downs in weight with an open mind, and if you can mentally accept these fluctuations, it will be easier to weigh yourself every morning and interpret the results clearly. So, how can you keep an open mind? If one morning your scales show an increase in your weight, don't get upset; instead, analyse it. Make a habit of doing a quick analysis each morning. Try to understand why your weight is up, down, or unchanged. This daily analysis will help you understand your previous day. What worked well? What did I eat yesterday that helped me stay within my calorie deficit, and did I enjoy that food? Was all my food throughout the day healthy and rich in protein? Did I have any snacks? If yes, were they managed and kept in small portions? If everything checks out, the final question is: Did I stick to my calorie deficit? If the morning weight is down or the same, I'd say you're doing something right. Try to repeat what you ate on another day for confirmation. If your weight is up, consider improving your food choices. I recommend checking your weight every morning, but if that makes you feel down, stop and do a weight check at least once a week. However, tracking your weight is essential to observe progress or setbacks in your journey.

As a helpful tip from me, it's excellent and very useful if your partner becomes your "partner in crime" on your journey to a better body. It works best if you both share similar goals and are on the same page. You can turn this into healthy competition between you two. Make it enjoyable by discussing it as a common topic daily. It can serve as a joint hobby that might also strengthen your relationship. From my own experience, it definitely improved my relationship.

Talking about healthy competition, I found a way to tease my lovely wife. Most digital scales give you all kinds of indicators based on your weight, height, body fat percentage, muscle mass, and other factors, but on my digital scale, at the bottom of all the indicators, it calculates your body age. It tells you the age of your body based on all measurements and how fit you are. If you are even a bit overweight, it will give you a body age the same as or more than your actual age, but if you are a fit person with a low body fat percentage and good muscle mass, your body age will be lower than your real age. I improved my body age significantly by losing weight and gaining muscle, and my body age decreased as well by dropping many years off my actual age. Playing the healthy competition card and teasing my wife, I mention to her that my digital scales show me that I'm twenty-three years old! So, very responsibly, I reminded her that she's in a relationship with a youngster. For her to be fit with good indicators, the digital scales were still showing a slightly higher body age than mine. So, she was on a mission to beat me and have a younger body age.

Magic Pill side-effects

Like any medication, the magic pill can have side effects. For each person, side effects can vary. Sometimes, pills work well, but for someone else, they may not, as we are different physically and mentally. Statistically, more than one in ten people experience side effects when using medication. These side effects can be very different for each individual, such as headache, dizziness, temperature, or vomiting, but the side effects of the magic pill are more like setbacks in your journey towards a perfect body. I would compare headache and dizziness to mood changes, your temperature to focusing on the wrong things, and vomiting to negative thoughts like, "Do I need to go through all these hard challenges?"

Let's take a closer look at each side effect, or what I like to call "fallbacks." One of the most common side effects of using medication is headache and dizziness, which are similar to mood swings. People's moods fluctuate just like their headaches, with both having moments of feeling up and down. When you experience persistent and severe headaches, you feel down and don't want to do anything. You just want to wrap yourself in a blanket and stay still. When the headache subsides, you feel relief, as if a heavy weight has been lifted from your shoulders. At that moment, you start to feel good and are ready to do things, but like everyone, you have mood swings from time to time, and you know that feeling when you're in a good mood, but in a split second, a bad one. These mood swings often happen because of different situations in your private life. When you're in a low mood, similar to having a headache, you can be easily distracted, so your goals tend to stay on the back burner, and you're the best reason can momentarily lose its effectiveness. For example, you'll often find that other people have contributed to your mood swings; they can easily cause your mood to spike or drop in an instant, but it's easy to blame others. In reality, it's you and your mind that influence your feelings.

Dizziness can feel quite strange; it might give you that odd, enjoyable sensation when it seems like the world is spinning. At the same time, this side effect can startle you and make you stop. This pause usually means staying still, grabbing something to hold onto, and waiting for nothing else to happen in that moment. Normally, when dizziness occurs, it lasts only a short while, but this moment of standstill forces you to pause and wait until things return to normal. Your mood is similar. When you're in a bad mood or no mood at all, you just want to stop for a moment before continuing. Sometimes, these activities may be important for reaching your goals. Having a low or bad mood can lead to setbacks, slowing your progress on your health journey. During these low moments, you often lose sight of your main motivation. It's difficult to lift yourself out of a low mood, but it is possible. All you need to do is focus on your priorities and goals. Remember the true reason you decided to change your life; remind yourself of your bigger picture in life and the reason that's worth dying for.

What about temperature as a side effect? Temperature-related side effects are more connected to physical rather than mental setbacks. Fever causes physical weakness and a sense of uselessness. When feeling weak, the first instinct for many is to give up quickly. However, side effects like a fever can be beneficial because when you have a temperature, your body is fighting something as a form of self-protection to survive and heal. Side effects like fever for your magic pill can sometimes even be necessary. Everyone experiences weakness from time to time, and it's easy to use it as an excuse to give up, but that only leads to failure or setbacks in pursuing your dreams. Side effects of a fever have two sides: negative and positive. Physical weakness is the dark side, but it's better to focus on the bright side. The bright side is your body's self-protection and healing system kicking in. My advice during such moments: take advantage of this self-protection. When you start losing focus on your goal, protect yourself by reminding yourself of what can change your life for the better, your magic pill, the best reason to get back on track and fight through weakness. Healing plays a vital role in this process. It is necessary for your recovery and to keep you moving forward. Its purpose is to help you restart the things you left behind. Everyone experiences setbacks; they are just a necessary part of your journey. Why are they necessary? Because success often requires failures or setbacks, which offer valuable lessons. Learning from mistakes helps you prepare for moments of pressure when you might feel like giving up. You'll learn what to do better or differently and what triggers your weakness and desire to give up without pressure. These are areas for improvement. For example, skipping your physical activities because you're tired after work and overthinking, like thinking, "My body needs rest, or I'll be useless at the gym today, so what's the point of going?" Then, you start to focus on the wrong reasons. So, what lesson can you learn, and what should you do differently to improve this? One option: find a visual reminder, like a picture of how you want to look, to motivate yourself. Remember, after good training, you will feel satisfied and proud of your effort. Another option: switch off your thinking for a moment. Don't think! Pack everything you need for your workout and just go! That's my favourite choice.

Fighting and dealing with weak moments will be challenging, but not if you are prepared and know what to expect and what you must do. Now, you will be more cautious about fallbacks, making it easier to overcome them. Remind yourself of your best reasons and their benefits.

None of the side effects is pleasant, but the worst of all is vomiting. Honestly, this side effect is tough. Vomiting brings a lot of mixed feelings. The feeling when it all comes out and it makes you feel sick straight away, then again causes cramps in your stomach, and just when you think it's over, it starts again. All the energy is drained from this relentless cycle. The only thing on your mind is to please stop. But what is vomiting as a side effect? It's when your body naturally tries to eliminate substances that could harm it. This returns to the body's self-protection mechanisms. In this case, your body is your mind, and the unwanted substance your mind wants to rid itself of is your new, non-comfort zone, your perfect body journey. It's possible that, with your magic pill, your mind may encounter this vomiting side effect at some point. Your mind attempts to protect you from anything outside your routine by rejecting new things. Your mind prefers to stay in its comfort zone, a lifestyle without stress, where everything is familiar and easy. But when something new appears outside that zone, and you feel unsure of what to do or how to proceed, your stress levels spike. This can lead to overthinking, questioning whether you need all this. These moments trigger your mind's self-protection mode, trying to purge new ideas through vomiting. It naturally happens to everyone from time to time. It might not happen immediately at the start of your journey towards a perfect body because you'll be full of excitement and motivation. However, sooner or later, it will occur. The key is to be prepared and learn how to handle this side effect. Thoughts like, 'Do I need all this?' or 'Why am I tormenting myself?' may arise. It's hard; is it worth it? You want more from life, so yes, it's worth it, and yes, you do need all that to become stronger. The secret is, it's all in your mind. Only you have the power to control these mental games. Learning how to take control of your mind is crucial – being in charge means you can win any battle. With every victory, you'll start to feel powerful, no matter what you do.

You only live once, so you should embrace it. There will be days or occasions that act as your fallbacks, which is good to have. You don't want to feel like a prisoner; you want to enjoy everything that life offers. Some days, you may skip calorie counting and simply enjoy food, or you might miss a day of exercise because of guilty pleasures like parties, BBQ weekends, or weddings, or even decide to treat your family to a meal out. Simple pleasures in life are essential for happiness, even if they set you back slightly on your journey to the perfect body; always remember to live and enjoy life. To maintain this journey and your new lifestyle, find activities you enjoy, such as making your diet enjoyable by including foods you love, but in smaller portions. Engage in physical activities that you genuinely want to do in your free time. Most importantly, live your life; indulge in guilty pleasures from time to time and accept the upcoming consequences. Be prepared, you might feel like you've taken a step back in your journey after one wild party weekend, but remember, this setback is only temporary. Don't panic; simply pick up where you left off before indulging in guilty pleasures. Be patient while your body recovers from these setbacks. Your mind will adapt more easily after experiencing your setbacks a few times. After these setbacks, you'll better understand how your body reacts, how quickly it gets back on track, and how you can best deal with the consequences. It's important to realise that while you pursue your ideal body and enjoy life, the main trade-off is that it will take longer to reach your goal. If you have a deadline for achieving your ideal body, I suggest limiting parties and exercising more discipline to stay focused on your key reasons.

I have my fallbacks, and I still indulge in guilty pleasures from time to time because I love myself and my life. During holidays, I don't stick to calorie counting or physical activity plans. Holidays are a time when I switch off from everything and recharge with fresh energy.

However, even on holiday, I catch myself unconsciously tracking calories and staying active. When you record all your calories, weigh every piece of food and drink, you learn how many calories are in each gram. There are staple foods you eat regularly, like standard breakfasts with two eggs, toast, and a hundred grams of mild pan-fried asparagus. As a new habit during breakfast preparation, weighing and recording your food, you'll know that one egg has around seventy calories, one medium toast about a hundred calories, and a hundred grams of asparagus has twenty calories, with a small amount of butter, say ten grams in the pan, adding around seventy calories to improve the asparagus's taste. So, for your breakfast, you'll have approximately three hundred thirty calories. If this is your usual breakfast, these numbers become embedded in your mind as basic food information. No matter where you are, whether it's a holiday, business trip, at home, or at a party with friends and family, you'll have these figures in your head. As I mentioned, I don't record my food during holidays, but when it's time to eat, I assess what I'll consume and intuitively estimate the grams and calories involved. The same applies to activities during a holiday. If you can't do your usual daily routines back home, explore your holiday destination on foot, walk around cities or places, and take part in fun activities like swimming or water sports. This way, you have fun while burning off those extra guilty pleasure calories. It's a win-win! Engaging in activities during your holiday also helps keep your body at a low-level target effortlessly. I'm a big fan of active holidays, and with such trips, I feel justified in treating myself to tasty food without overthinking it. Everyone has their own idea of a holiday, but extra steps, enjoyable activities, and fresh air never hurt your journey to a perfect body. They also help you mentally switch off or clear your mind. Spending at least half of your holiday days engaged in fun activities is healthier than spending the entire week sitting in front of a pool with little movement. Don't get me wrong, time by the pool is also necessary; it offers good recovery after a busy, active, and fun-filled day. And why not treat yourself to some peace and relaxation beside the pool after an active day filled with fun?

Back from holiday and back to reality. You're back in your morning routine, stepping onto your scales. You see, your weight has increased. Your body fat percentage is also up. Your first reaction might be disappointment and panic. That's it! The sky is falling! Seeing those high numbers on your scales, you might feel ready to give up. All your hard work seems to have gone out of the window! Inside, you get that feeling of breaking apart, you want to cry, scream, shout, and swear! Wait, this person is no longer you! The new you is positive, with a smile on your face, calm and confident, knowing and already expecting these results. In a short while, you will be back where you left off. Just stick to strict discipline, and you will see results. By keeping an open mind and accepting the possibility of high numbers, you'll avoid the shock and setbacks that could derail your motivation and progress. With your mind prepared for what's ahead, you'll be in a better position to pick up where you left off.

Previously, I talked about your best reason, your magic pill. A pill that motivates you and helps you achieve your dreams, a pill that works wonders. But how about a different story? How about the best reasons not to do something? One of your side effects will be excuses, reasons why not to do this. Excuses can be very powerful because they can be both the best and worst at the same time. It is important to turn all negative reasons into positive ones. Remember, not all excuses seem negative, but a simple excuse can have negative side effects. I'll give an example I mentioned before. I'll start working on my perfect body on the first of January! Great, but it's September! Your New Year's resolution is set, and there's nothing negative about this idea; however, waiting for the perfect day to start working on your perfect body will give you more time to come up with more excuses - reasons not to do it! In four months, many things can happen, and most importantly, you can lose the true power of that magic pill. The best reason worth dying for can change and may no longer be the best reason after a month. If you have your perfect reason, act immediately to stay motivated for achievement. It's a perfect example of how a great idea can have unintended side effects when starting your journey. In this case, don't wait for the perfect day; create one!

Those days when you just can't be bothered, or when you're changing your fitness plans, like being ready to skip your physical activity session. I can guarantee one hundred percent that you'll have those moments, but now you will be prepared for them. So, what do you need to succeed in your routine? Your recipe for success will be set for days and times. When you have a fixed plan for what you do on specific days and times, and everyone around you knows about it, you'll have fewer excuses to skip them. It will become your new fixed routine, your new lifestyle. Sticking with that routine over time, you'll start to be proud of it. For negative possibilities, you'll be prepared by transforming something negative into a positive. It's not always black and white; your negative may be clear in this case, but there can be something positive in the setup of a strict routine. Always try to see the bigger picture. Sometimes it's not about a literal positive element, but it can lead to a positive outcome. Those negative and tempting reasons often put people in a situation where they need to choose to go right or left, tempted to find a reason why not to stick with their best reason. That little devil on your left shoulder will tell you to go left, to make your life easier, which always sounds the most attractive. The left route will be filled with countless reasons of "why not". Most people's first instinct is to make excuses or find reasons to avoid all hard things and obstacles! We, as humans, are weak and tend to say no more often than yes. To be lazy, we like to find reasons not to do things, and we are always waiting for a better time, weather, or situation. Don't wait for the 1st of January to start working towards your perfect body. Do it today; find your best reason, don't wait, use it now so it can kick in by tomorrow. Don't wait for some special day; don't make excuses. Break that chain of excuses holding you back from starting or returning to your ideal body goal. Starting or restarting your journey on a day without significance can be incredibly powerful. Just an ordinary day, without reason, will make you feel one step closer to your goal. With that step, you break the chain of your first excuse to postpone starting. Now, this day without meaning will become a day with one of the greatest meanings in your life. How often in life do we have special days worth remembering and being proud of? Be proud of every small achievement, and don't choose the easy way out. Challenge yourself to avoid the left route to strengthen your mind.

The right path will always be the hardest, with no excuses. This decision begins with no reason to make excuses. This path will present obstacles throughout, but by controlling your mind, you will fight, sacrifice, and learn how to manage all these negative thoughts and excuses. With belief and confidence, you will push through to the end of this tough journey because you know you have secured the realisation of your dream at the end of your perfect body journey. People will admire you for these qualities. They will see you as a stronger person, both physically and mentally, and that will motivate you further. Having that increased confidence and drive, you will be even more motivated to achieve your promised goals and new ones.

The consequences, my favourite topic. The basics of not sticking to your plan will lead you back to where you started, or even worse, and then you will believe that nothing works for you. The simple secret to avoiding failure is to have a plan and stick to it consistently. No matter what the situation, I always consider the potential consequences. For me, it's easy because, for as long as I can remember, I have always thought first and then acted. That's probably the reason why I've been blessed with fewer problems in my life. Seeing and realising the consequences before making any decision can have a significant impact on your life, making things much easier, reducing stress, and allowing you to focus on the right things.

What possible consequences can arise if you decide to switch off completely during your holiday? The answer is: not many, but this approach will only work if you are mentally strong enough to see a fallback and realise it's only temporary. There are always consequences, whether good or bad, positive or negative, but if you are mentally prepared for them and have a plan in place, you'll be in a better position. Problems begin when a person cannot process negative consequences; for example, seeing significant weight gain after a wonderful holiday. With amazing and positive emotions on the first day back, you step on the scales and see your weight has increased. This number on the scale was that high two months ago. It's easy to get upset because a week's holiday ruins two months' hard work. If you don't get a grip on your mind and lose control, allowing feelings to take over, it can be devastating. Many people give up as a result. People often feel defeated and demotivated because they work hard to achieve their ideal body and have been punished for wanting to enjoy their lives. It seems you can't want both, but I disagree. That's perfectly fine; you can have and do both! You can live your life and still strive for your ideal body. The key to handling this consequence lies in your mindset. Before stepping on the scales, you must be willing to accept that higher weight number from two or even three months ago. Being prepared to confront that will help you absorb the shock. Knowing there's a way to return to just before holiday weight will make you feel less stressed and keep your motivation alive. You've seen before that it works, and now it will work again, so step on the scales with a smile and full confidence. There will always be consequences. Consider what could go wrong, whether you can handle it, and if you're okay with it, then live your life.

The pill did magic! What next?

Congratulations, you've achieved your perfect body!

It would be wonderful to skip all previous chapters and jump directly into this one. In real life, we know that's not possible, and there's a reason for that. Most people have very destructive habits. These habits often lead to losing what they have. If you can obtain something without fighting for it or wanting it excessively, it will quickly lose value once you get it. There's a saying, "easy come, easy go." Today, most material things are so easy to acquire that people simply want them and go out to get them, but soon after, they desire something new. A perfect example is mobile phones. Nowadays, you just go and get the latest model; when the next one comes out, people rush to change without any real reason, just because they can. In my young adult years, life taught me to want and dream for a long time before I finally got my dream phone. I dreamt about that phone day and night, imagining myself holding it. When I finally had it, I felt so proud because I had achieved one of my dreams at that moment. My magic pill for that moment was to have something cool that only I possessed, something that would make my friends admire me, like a confidence boost. In my youth, most people value material possessions and believe that having all the cool, expensive things makes you someone important, but as we know, true values lie elsewhere. I sent many signals to the universe expressing my readiness for that phone. I waited patiently, saved money, and truly desired it. When I got it, I didn't even consider upgrading to a newer model because I had wanted that phone for so long. I kept it for three years until the microphone stopped working, and the battery only lasted four hours without charging. The last month with that phone, barely hearing what people said during calls and constantly searching for a charger every four hours, was not enjoyable at all. So, I had good reasons and a suitable moment to replace my dream phone with a new one. This was a repeated cycle of desire building up and then struggling to appreciate what I already had. What I want to say is that if you can achieve your ideal body very quickly, you won't appreciate it and will lose it just as fast because you won't see its true value. Conversely, going through the process allows you to cherish every small achievement. You will value each step of your journey, every drop of sweat, and every internal fight you face to reach your goal. All your accomplishments will retain their worth, helping you to maintain or even improve the goals you have already attained. It should prevent you from reverting to old habits or an unwanted lifestyle.

This chapter is a moment in your life that will feel like a bonus for all your hard work. That moment when you reach your goal will be a mixed one because, at that point, you will have developed strong mental and physical resilience. You've tested what it means to be ambitious and how to achieve each small goal along the way. The mixed feelings of excitement for your big goal and the sensation that nothing special is happening will come from you, as you will have so many new ideas of what to do and achieve. Your mind will feel like nothing can stop you; if you can achieve this, you can do anything.

Back to the main goal: your perfect body. When you reach the point of achieving the perfect body look, you will start to think, "If I've come this far, I can do better." Now you have a choice about what to do next. From all this perfect body experience, you gain powerful tools. No matter what your next step for the future is, you will need your next magic pill. Let's be honest, you will want the next magic pill because, as I said, you will be addicted to the success from that magic.

So, we know this pill works wonders! What's next? First, you could enhance your already perfect body for an even better appearance, but you'll need a new reason to do so. Once you have your new magic pill, develop a new plan. Create a fresh routine, modify your diet, adjust your calorie intake, and change your habits if necessary. Do everything you have done so far to reach this point.

The second option would be to maintain your already perfect body. That could mean you're content with what you have and what you've achieved, so now it's a new you. That's great, congratulations, you deserve it! Along with that comes an appreciation of the hard work you've put into reaching your goal. Remember to value every step of your journey to sustain what you have and what you've worked for. If you choose this second option, you'll have a small treat. You can indulge in a bit more food. Only a bit more! Just don't revert to old habits. You still need to stick to the daily calorie allowance. The good news is, you won't see this as a problem, as being on a tight calorie deficit will become normal for your mind. It will become second nature. You will understand how many calories are in every piece of food, how much you can eat, when to indulge a little, and when to avoid it. After doing this for a long time, you've trained yourself to see it as a normal daily activity, like writing, reading, talking, or breathing. Remember, to maintain your perfect body, you no longer need to be in a calorie deficit. Your life can now become a bit easier. You can add roughly a couple of hundred calories on top of your previous daily intake, and that could be your maintenance calorie level. I suggest you check and test what number of calories works best for maintaining your perfect body, as this can vary from person to person. Nowadays, we have excellent online tools. Simply type "Calorie maintenance calculator" into any search engine and determine your new calorie target as a guide for maintenance. Test these new calories for two or three months, and stay consistent, as you were before, to see the best results. Don't forget to monitor your body fat percentage, as it is your key indicator. Aim to keep your body fat percentage low. The goal is to find your comfort zone. Adjust your calories gradually until they fit and work for you in the long run. Just give your body time to adapt to the new changes. Find what suits you best and stick with it. You will experience that incredible feeling of freedom.

Now, there is a bit of a problem! As an ambitious person, choosing the first option to set new challenges and new goals will work very well for you because your mind will be busier focusing on new objectives. However, for ambitious people, the nice problem to have is that when you achieve your goal, you need the next goal in your life. The issue starts when you are happy with your perfect body and decide to stick with the second choice. This choice lacks the next big step: what comes next? If you only have some other things going on in your life, you might feel a bit lost. Only a small number of people will probably have this problem, but if you are one of them, remember this: at the point when you achieve your goal and feel a bit lost and don't understand what's happening, and can't find your place, and inside, something is dragging you crazy, the solution is simple. Find the next thing, keep driving yourself for new improvements, and make yourself the best version you can be. Be addicted to your magic pills for a better you.

Let me tell you, the most annoying question related to this chapter was what people kept asking throughout my perfect body journey, from the moment they found out about my goal to achieving a six-pack and sculpting my ideal physique. I've been asked the same silly question repeatedly: "What will you do when you reach your goal?" I never understood the point of this question or what people expected me to say. I hated this question! I've never heard anyone ask this silly question to someone whose goal is to quit smoking. Like, what will you do when you quit smoking? Of course, the goal is quitting smoking, but the main aim is never to smoke again, and it's the same in this case. When you achieve your perfect body goal, you will no longer want your old, unwanted body. After being asked this silly question a few times, I came up with a standard answer. I'd have two options: maintain or improve, but the main thing is to stay fit and never go back!

The truth is, you need to plant a seed in your mind: my life will be different from the day I begin my journey to achieve the perfect body. And let's be honest, you don't want to go through all this challenging, hard work only to throw it all away in the end because of old, tempting, lazy lifestyle habits. Only halfway through my journey, when my commitment to my goal was rock solid, I realised that this has become my new lifestyle and it will be mine forever.

This new, ambitious lifestyle, this new you with a perfect body, should be and will be a lifelong commitment! It's important to understand that if you begin this journey, you must stay with it and create a new you for life. After years, you can look back and reflect on how difficult it was and how much you have transformed your life. I wish you to be healthy, confident, successful, and passionate about life. Just want it!

Summary

So, now you are in the final chapter of this book, and I hope you are still eager for changes in your life. No more feeling unfit; no more hiding behind excuses. With all the information in this book, you have plenty of thinking and analysing to do. As you read through it, I wish you could see yourself from the side view, and I hope you have done it. It will offer an opportunity to step out of your usual life routine. Using the life examples provided in this book, try to picture yourself for a better understanding of where you may be lacking or making mistakes and how to change them to be where you want to be. I suppose the goal is a healthier lifestyle? Take a moment to reflect on yourself and aim for greatness. Consider what habits and actions worked for you and what you would never do again. With this magic pill and some changes, you can lead a completely different lifestyle where you are confident, successful, healthy, and have the impressive physique you desire.

The Magic Pill. A solution for all your problems. We are all so tired of trying and failing, feeling exhausted and longing for just this one magical pill. A pill we can obtain somewhere and swallow to let the magic do everything for us. Just by having this pill, your life will change. And now you have the magic pill. Maybe not exactly how you expected it to look, but it makes sense. Your best reason for what it takes to succeed will get you to any goal you wish. For example, every successful person who comes to mind, whether the fitness influencers you follow with their perfect bodies or just a successful friend or family member, all had the best reason to be where they are now. They had this magic pill, the best reason to drive and achieve their goals.

Imagine how strong and how many magic pills the richest person in the world has? This person probably had more than one magic pill to become a billionaire. But it started with one reason, which could be something simple like, "I'll prove them wrong," or "I'll prove I can be successful!" Only this person knows the real reason that pushed them towards unbelievable success. It always begins with one strong reason, but throughout the journey, you gather more and more reasons. When you feel that taste of success, you know it's working, and you start becoming addicted to this magic pill of success.

This book is a guide to your perfect body. But is it really? As you read through chapter after chapter, you will begin to realise that this book offers much more than just a way to achieve your perfect body. It provides endless possibilities and shares insights into common problems across various, yet similar, areas of life. You might recognise some familiar examples from your own experiences. This is a bonus because if you already know the answers to your problems, fixing them should be easier, right? There are things you didn't know and elements you've never had, things that are missing for your success. For example, the most important thing to have is "the best reason that's worth dying for", the reason that will passionately drive you to achieve any success. Let's examine the opposite side of absence, ignorance, and inaction regarding goal achievement. These are the actions you take, but often for the wrong reasons. It's vital to recognise how you may be unconsciously stopping yourself from reaching your dreams through repetitive mistakes. The things you keep getting wrong trap you in a cycle that can be hard to break free from. Nevertheless, you have all the answers; the only thing you need to do is take action to resolve your problems and succeed in any area of your life. This book provides eye-opening insights: if your mind is in the right place and motivated by the right reasons, there are no limits for you.

Each chapter has been designed for your learning. I'll summarise the key information you need from each chapter to maximise your understanding and learning.

The first chapter will help you recognise when enough is enough. You must admit you have a problem, and while it's not too late, you need to do something about it. However, you feel tired of trying and failing, just desperately wishing for a magic pill to fix your ongoing issues, and here I am, telling you that there is a magic pill for your problems. Of course, nothing in this world is free, and I'm not talking about needing to pay money to buy this magic pill. I'm saying that you will need to take action to get this pill. Like any medicine, when you need it, you must do your part to obtain it. Be prepared to put in effort and take action to get this magic pill, and also be ready for a bumpy ride since it's part of the journey.

The second chapter poses a question. Are you the right person for the magic pill? I mention situations and examples from life for you to compare and analyse. This chapter is all about stopping and thinking. These examples help you imagine yourself in these situations to understand what you may have done wrong and what you haven't done to be successful so far. Additionally, I present some habits that naturally prevent us from achieving success. Only you can decide whether you will succeed or not, but some effort will be necessary from you. So, are you the right person for the magic pill? The answer to this question is: Yes! You deserve a magic pill to make your life more enjoyable, to achieve success, and to be happy with yourself.

In the third chapter, I aim to help you build trust in me. To earn your trust, I shared some personal stories and experiences from my life. What I've shared is very personal, but let's be honest: the problems, solutions, and journey to a perfect body will be relatable to everyone. I'm one of you; I've been where you are now. I am an ordinary person living a family life with a standard nine-to-five, five-day work week. I faced the same problems and insecurities as many others, but I found answers and solutions. With a positive and open mindset, I hope your trust will encourage you to go for this magic pill and give it a try for yourself.

And there it is, the fourth chapter. You finally discover what this magical pill is, where to get it, and what you need to do to experience its magic. I hope you won't be disappointed, but rather relieved to understand what was missing for success. You only need one thing to start your journey. **"The best reason that's worth dying for!"** In this chapter, I'll give examples of what motivates most people and what can be a perfect and strong reason for dreams to come true. The life-changing benefits that people can gain from having the right priorities and reasons in their lives. This magic pill can be more than just a way to achieve your perfect body; it can also lead to success in many other areas of your life. Taking control of your mind opens up many new possibilities and makes you feel powerful and successful. Keeping an open mind will change the way we think, leading to a sense that anything is possible. We all have at least one magic pill; the only difference is that successful people have found it, and from this one pill, they generate more because they have a taste of success. For each person, success means something different, but witnessing major achievements is a perfect example of the power of the magic pill. Achievements like being the richest person in the world, or people who can run distances that seem impossible, those who fail hundreds of times inventing new, seemingly impossible things for our mind, or simply the power of this pill can encourage successful individuals to change their lifestyles from stressful lives to one of happiness and peace, away from everyone. They all have at least one good reason for where they are, with their success. For this reason, combined with taking charge of your mind, you will have everything you need to achieve your dreams.

Now that you know what this magic pill is and understand what you need, I want to offer some extra help to put you in a better position to achieve your dreams. For some people, a perfect reason might be enough, but for most, extra assistance is necessary. In this chapter, you will find a recipe for your reason supported by a double-strength supplement. Your goal will be much easier to reach if you establish good habits in your daily routine, and it all begins with discipline. On your journey to achieving your ideal body, elements such as setting smart goals, developing healthy habits, maintaining a positive mindset, and adopting a healthy, stress-free lifestyle will make the process much simpler. People often jump straight to the main goal, but they frequently forget to organise everything around them. Living without all the essential vitamins and nutrients can lead to failure because there are too many distractions and daily problems to handle, constantly pushing you off track and preventing you from reaching your goals. Use this double-strength recipe to eliminate all excuses and prevent yourself from failing.

Positive addictions are a good problem to have! Being addicted to success means you know what you need for your dreams to come true, which will make you look and feel more confident. Love your body and use it as a benchmark to love yourself even more. In this chapter, I want to dare you to embrace these new benefits without fear. People will start to see you differently, as someone they want to keep close for good advice or whom they can trust to get things done; it's part of success. Achieve your perfect body, feel successful, and then embrace confidence. And that's how addiction in this case will look and feel.

In the next chapter, you will discover which three types of people you are. These three types offer some clarity to help you avoid failure. Since you are reading this book and have come this far, it is clear to me which type you belong to, if only you take the time to think this through and clarify your priorities. Be honest with yourself to prevent feelings of failure.

How to swallow a pill? At this point in the book, you will have some essential information and actions that are crucial for success. You will find the basic guidance to help you progress and all the essentials you need to lose body fat. The magic pill works wonders, but for magic to happen, you must follow certain actions and steps towards achieving your perfect body goal and realising your dreams. Follow the steps and ensure necessary things are in place so you don't feel like you are doing something extra to reach your goal. Always, at the beginning, you need to put in some effort and take additional actions, but over time, it will become a part of your standard routine. You will learn to train your mind and take control of it.

You should be aware that there will be some setbacks on your journey to achieving the perfect body. Like most pills, certain side effects are to be expected. During your journey, you will face challenging moments, but with the right motivation and a positive mindset, these moments are manageable, and in a short time, you can regain your momentum towards your goals.

Achieving your ideal body goal will open a new chapter for you, a new lifestyle from now on, lasting forever. All hard work and sacrifices should be appreciated. At this point, the world is accessible to you, and you will feel capable of doing and achieving everything because you have accomplished the most challenging goal. Never revert to old habits. Live life with your newly loved body and cherished lifestyle. Be proud of who you have become.

After reading this book, please don't put it away; keep it nearby so you can easily refer to it from time to time for a refreshing boost or to rediscover forgotten answers. Only you can create change, but to do so, you must desire it so intensely that you become the best motivation for overcoming any obstacle. Most importantly, you need to take action on your problem because, as people, we often wait with hope that something will happen and things will sort themselves out, but that's not always the case. If you want something, you have to go and get it yourself. Find your best reason for your goal and use it whenever you feel the need to boost yourself. I always ask myself: what's the worst thing that can happen if I try? So, ask yourself the same question: what's the worst thing that could happen if I try to follow this book's tips, tricks, and ideas? Everyone can do it, so can you!

Your perfect body, not the one on magazine covers, but the body where you feel your best, so you can feel free and enjoy your life.

Remember, your "magic pill" is your
"THE BEST REASON THAT'S WORTH DYING FOR."

Disclaimer

This book is written for informational, educational, and motivational purposes only. Here, I, as the author, offer my personal perspective. Drawing on years of experience, ideas, and my own opinions about weight loss, fitness, health, personal development, relationships, and mindset, I am not providing any medical, psychological, nutritional, or other professional advice. Always consult a qualified professional before beginning any new programme, as dietary and exercise changes can significantly affect your life and lifestyle. The main focus of this book is "the right reason", the motivation to achieve a healthier and better-looking body by following some ideas and tasks; however, no guarantees are made regarding weight loss, body transformation, mental well-being, or any other specific results. Every individual is different, and various factors can influence results. The concept of the "perfect body" varies from person to person; there is no promise of achieving any specific physical or aesthetic outcome. Topics such as relationships, motivation, emotional patterns, and mental blocks are included to encourage self-reflection and awareness only. These topics are not intended to diagnose, treat, or cure any mental health conditions. By reading this book, you acknowledge that you are fully responsible for your own actions, decisions, and outcomes. I, as the author, shall not be held liable for any damage, physical, mental, or emotional injury, loss, or otherwise that may occur directly or indirectly from the information contained within the book. This book is provided "as is" without warranties of any kind and is intended for a global audience.

www.ingramcontent.com/pod-product-compliance
Lightning Source LLC
Chambersburg PA
CBHW070030040426
42333CB00040B/1419